Dental
Assisting
Exam
Preparation

Dental Assisting Exam Preparation

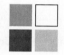

Hazel O. Torres, CDA, RDA, RDAEF, MA
Formerly Director, Dental Assisting
College of Marin
Kentfield, California

Lois E. Mazzucchi-Ballard, CDA, RDA, MA
Formerly Director, Dental Assisting
Santa Rosa Junior College
Santa Rosa, California

W.B. SAUNDERS COMPANY
A Division of Harcourt Brace & Company
Philadelphia   London   Toronto   Montreal   Sydney   Tokyo

W.B. Saunders Company
A Division of Harcourt Brace & Company

The Curtis Center
Independence Square West
Philadelphia, Pennsylvania 19106

Library of Congress Cataloging-in-Publication Data

Torres, Hazel O.
    Dental assisting exam preparation / Hazel O. Torres, Lois E. Mazzucchi-Ballard.

    1. Dental assistants — Examinations, questions, etc.   2. Dentistry — Examinations, questions, etc.   I. Mazzucchi-Ballard, Lois E.   II. Title.
    [DNLM: 1. Dental Assistants — examination questions.   2. Dental Care — examination questions.   WU 18.5 T693d 1994]
    RK60.5.T669 1994
    617.6′0233′076 — dc20
    DNLM/DLC   93-19477

DENTAL ASSISTING EXAM PREPARATION   ISBN 0-7216-3295-5

Printed in The United States of America.

Last digit is the print number: 10   9   8   7   6   5   4   3   2

We dedicate this book, Dental Assisting Exam Preparation,
to the memory of Murray L. Ballard, DDS, and Carl L. Torres.
These gentlemen were steadfast in their support
of our efforts in dental auxiliary education and
particularly the dental assisting profession
throughout many years.

Dental Assisting Exam Preparation

Preface

This book has been designed to help candidates prepare for the Dental Assisting National Board or for licensure examinations for dental assistants administered by individual states.

Included are three comprehensive tests, two on general chairside functions and one on dental radiography. These tests closely follow the format of the examinations cited above. The questions are multiple choice, matching, pictorial, and fill-in. They are task-oriented to give the candidate an opportunity to demonstrate an understanding of the functions performed, rather than just the ability to recall details.

Graduates of accredited dental assisting programs, and those applicants for certification or state licensure who have met eligibility requirements by way of another route will profit from taking these examinations and comparing their answers with answers presented by the authors, which are provided with explanatory information.

Individuals are encouraged to approach the examinations as they would the formal tests by the independent agencies mentioned above. If the candidate is unsuccessful in the first trial test, it is advised that a period of study take place, particularly in areas where insufficient knowledge has been demonstrated, before the second trial test is taken. It is further expected that a candidate will attempt these tests in the same formal atmosphere as would be experienced when the actual licensure and certification examinations are administered.

The topics for questions on these review tests include the following:

- Protocol for infection control
- Basic sciences as related to anatomy and physiology
- The collection and recording of clinical data related to oral conditions and general health screening
- Dental radiography; clinical techniques and integrated health and safety factors
- Clinical chairside and laboratory procedures in the general and specialty practices of dentistry, including armamentarium, materials, anesthesia, and medications
- Patient education, including nutrition as well as other forms of oral health management
- Prevention and management of medical and dental emergencies to include pharmacology
- Dental office management

Because all of these examinations are task-oriented, the candidate is encouraged to study and review all categories of information with the intent to recognize reasons, causes, effects, and symptoms that direct a particular action.

A comprehensive reference list is included in the text to assist candidates in seeking additional information to enhance their knowledge of a particular subject.

Hazel O. Torres
Lois E. Mazzucchi-Ballard

Contents

INTRODUCTION

As has been noted in the Preface, this text has been developed to help a candidate prepare for the Dental Assisting National Board Examination for certification and for licensure and registration as a dental assistant in the individual states. The ability to answer 75 percent of these test questions should ensure that the candidate has the basic knowledge of the subject matter covered to successfully answer related questions found on the national or state examinations.

To maximize the benefits of sitting for each of the three examinations offered in this text, a candidate should approach each as he or she would in the classroom or when actually sitting for a board examination and realize that an honest evaluation of the results must follow. The percentage of correct and incorrect answers should be noted, as well as where additional knowledge is needed.

It is recommended that each test be removed from the book, assembled, and stapled before proceeding. The authors' answer sheets should not be reviewed until an entire test has been completed, and they then should be attached to the test papers for easy reference at any future time.

At least 3 hours of uninterrupted time should be allowed for each of the first two tests, and at least 2 hours for the radiology examination. A candidate should be physically comfortable and free of distractions. All printed instructions should be read in their entirety so that the correct format is selected. Each question should also be carefully read in its entirety before an attempt is made to answer it. There should be no confusion about what is actually being asked.

Most multiple choice questions contain at least one distractor that appears to be just as valid as the correct answer. The BEST answer should always be selected. It is not wise to labor too long on a difficult question, for this can cause unnecessary frustration. Instead, mark the problem question and return to it when the others have been answered.

The authors' answer sheets, which are found in a separate section of the book, should be referred to after completion of a test. They frequently offer, in addition to the correct answer, background information on the subject or an explanation of why a particular answer is correct or incorrect.

If, after correcting his or her answers to the first review test, a candidate finds a definite weakness in a given area, it is suggested that, in addition to studying the answer sheet, a textbook be studied for more complete information until the candidate is entirely comfortable with his or her command of that subject matter. The candidate should then proceed to Test II, treating it in the same professional manner as Test I. The Radiology Examination may then be undertaken, again following the procedure described earlier. Candidates should remember that to profit from these review tests,

1

they must be entirely honest when evaluating their test results and the amount of review needed.

These review examinations have been developed with basic objectives in mind. They are based on the functions and related knowledge necessary for a certified, registered, licensed, or expanded function dental assistant to serve as a responsible member of the dental health team and to meet the criteria established by the dental practice acts of the various states for the delegation and supervision of functions.

In 1990, the American Dental Association published *Legal Provisions for Delegating Functions to Dental Assistants and Dental Hygienists*. However, provisions may have changed since then, so the authors suggest that persons seeking information about the provisions of an individual state contact the state's dental governing board to obtain a copy of the current dental practice act. A request should also be made to receive a list of delegatable functions for a dental assistant's performance, along with the level of supervision required by dentists in the particular state where the candidate resides.

GOOD LUCK.

TEST I

General Dental Assisting

TEST 1

1. A patient's health history MUST include what essential facts in order to plan a dental treatment schedule?

① most recent exposure to ionizing radiation
② allergies and sensitivities
③ routine medication
④ change in health habits
⑤ current nutritional pattern

    ⓐ 1, 3
    ⓑ 2, 4
    ⓒ 1, 2, 3
    ⓓ 2, 3, 5
    ⓔ all of the above

2. A patient's diagnostic signs include which of the following?

① respiration rate
② pulse
③ temperature
④ blood pressure
⑤ weight

    ⓐ 1, 2, 3
    ⓑ 1, 2, 3, 4
    ⓒ 2, 3, 5
    ⓓ 1, 2, 4, 5

3. A patient's pulse rate is measured and recorded as

    ⓐ impulses

    ⓑ systolic rate

    ⓒ diastolic rate

    ⓓ beats per minute

4. A patient's blood pressure is primarily monitored by placing a cuff and stethoscope on the

    ⓐ jugular vein

    ⓑ brachial artery

    ⓒ facial vein

    ⓓ radial artery

5. Average adult blood pressure is

    ⓐ 120 systolic/70 diastolic

    ⓑ 120 diastolic/60 systolic

    ⓒ 95 systolic/60 diastolic

    ⓓ 95 diastolic/70 systolic

6. The normal respiration rate for a woman is approximately how many breaths per minute?

    ⓐ 12

    ⓑ 14

    ⓒ 16

    ⓓ 18

7. Which of the following procedures should be followed to prevent cross-contamination when obtaining a patient's temperature?

    ① disinfect the thermometer

    ② store the thermometer in a sterile container

    ③ place a disposable sleeve over the thermometer

    ④ provide the patient with antiseptic mouthwash

    ⓐ 1, 3

    ⓑ 1, 4

    ⓒ 1, 2, 3

    ⓓ 2, 4

8. To ensure an accurate temperature reading, an oral mercury thermometer should be
   1. held at the bulb end
   2. held parallel to the floor
   3. turned slowly to view extension of mercury
   4. read immediately

   a. 1, 3
   b. 2, 4
   c. 1, 2, 3
   d. 2, 3, 4

9. A clinical examination of the hard and soft tissues of a patient's intraoral cavity includes which of the following structures?
   1. the buccal mucosa
   2. the commissures of the lips
   3. the tongue
   4. the palate
   5. the oropharynx and uvula

   a. 1, 2, 3
   b. 1, 3, 4
   c. 1, 3, 4, 5
   d. 2, 3, 4

10. Which of the following are included in a clinical examination of a dental patient's extraoral soft tissues?
    1. gentle kneading of the lips
    2. palpation of the nares
    3. examination of the philtrum and the vermilion border
    4. examination of the labial frenum attachment

    a. 1, 3
    b. 2, 4
    c. 2, 3, 4
    d. all of the above

11. Which of the following are benign exostoses of the oral cavity?
    1. palatal rugae
    2. torus mandibularis
    3. retromolar pad
    4. torus palatinus

Continued on next page

(a) 1, 3

(b) 1, 4

(c) 2, 3

(d) 2, 4

12. Any closed epithelium-lined cavity or sac usually containing liquid or semisolid material is

(a) an abscess

(b) a vesicle

(c) a cyst

(d) a pustule

13. When updating a patient's health history, a dental assistant must request additional information in regard to which medications?

1 home remedies

2 over-the-counter drugs

3 topical applications

4 prescription medications

(a) 1, 2, 3

(b) 1, 2, 4

(c) 2, 3, 4

(d) 1, 2, 3, 4

14. A dentist who dispenses drugs to patients is required to keep accurate records of

1 controlled substances purchased

2 controlled substances dispensed

3 prescriptions written

4 remedies advised

5 analgesics purchased

(a) 1, 2, 3

(b) 1, 2, 4

(c) 2, 3, 4

(d) all of the above

15. If two drugs have a *synergistic* relationship, it means that

(a) they are incompatible

(b) they are compatible

ⓒ when taken together, one drug reduces the effectiveness of the other

ⓓ when taken together, the effects of the two drugs are enhanced

16. Patients with a history of angina pectoris may carry what medication with them to place under their tongue in case of an attack?

ⓐ amphetamine

ⓑ morphine

ⓒ nitroglycerin

ⓓ aspirin with codeine

17. To disinfect alginate or elastomer impressions before they are sent to a laboratory technician, the impression is sprayed with

ⓐ 2 percent glutaraldehyde solution

ⓑ iodophor solution

ⓒ isopropyl alcohol

ⓓ a, b

ⓔ a, c

18. To ensure a homogeneous mix of Rubberloid type elastomeric impression pastes, the first step is to

ⓐ spread the base paste on a cool, dry glass slab and let it stand for 15 seconds

ⓑ place catalyst paste on the stainless steel spatula

ⓒ spread the catalyst paste on the base paste and let it stand for 15 seconds before continuing the mix

ⓓ spread the base paste on the catalyst paste and let it stand for 15 seconds before continuing the mix

19. Which of the following is indicated when placing copal varnish on the dentin of a prepared tooth?

① one coat minimum

② one coat maximum

③ four coats maximum

④ two coats minimum

ⓐ 1, 2

ⓑ 2, 4

ⓒ 1, 3

ⓓ 4 only

20. The criteria for mixing dental cements for bases or for luting cast restorations include using a glass slab of

    (a) high temperature

    (b) low temperature

    (c) temperature below the dew point

    (d) temperature above the dew point

21. The amount of cement powder that can be incorporated into the cement liquid can be reduced by

    (1) a cool, dry glass slab

    (2) a warm, dry glass slab

    (3) slow spatulation of the mix

    (4) rapid spatulation of the mix

        (a) 1, 3

        (b) 2, 3

        (c) 2, 4

        (d) 4 only

22. Which of the following anticariogenic agents is present in several current dental cements?

    (a) phosphoric acid

    (b) chloroform

    (c) alumina

    (d) fluoride

23. Which of the following ingredients prevents zinc phosphate cement from adhering to the placement instrument?

    (a) cement powder

    (b) isopropyl 70 percent alcohol

    (c) eight volume hydrogen peroxide

    (d) bicarbonate of soda

24. The instrumentation and mixing procedure for ethoxybenzoic acid (EBA) cement is similar to mixing

    (a) zinc oxide – eugenol

    (b) calcium hydroxide

    (c) zinc phosphate

    (d) glass ionomer

25. An automixer dispenser for vinyl polysiloxane-type impression material moves the plunger forward to force the

① base and accelerator from the individual chambers
② pastes into the mixing tip
③ materials to blend and exit the tip as a uniform paste
④ catalyst ahead of the base material

ⓐ 1, 2
ⓑ 1, 3
ⓒ 1, 2, 3
ⓓ 4 only

26. To prevent sensitivity in a newly restored tooth, a dental assistant should

ⓐ thoroughly dry the dentin
ⓑ use cold air in the preparation
ⓒ use hot air in the preparation
ⓓ avoid desiccating the dentin

27. Directions for mixing glass ionomer cement for luting designate what ratio of powder to liquid?

① one scoop powder
② three scoops powder
③ two drops liquid
④ four drops liquid

ⓐ 1, 2
ⓑ 1, 3
ⓒ 2, 3
ⓓ 2, 4

28. The mix of glass ionomer cement for a luting procedure is accomplished in a

ⓐ minimum of 10 seconds
ⓑ maximum of 20 seconds
ⓒ minimum of 30 seconds
ⓓ maximum of 40 seconds

29. The ratio of glass ionomer cement powder to liquid for Class III and Class V restorations is

① one scoop of powder
② two scoops of powder

Continued on next page

③ one drop of liquid

④ three drops of liquid

    ⓐ 1, 3

    ⓑ 1, 4

    ⓒ 2, 3

    ⓓ 2, 4

30. The dental cement compatible with all restorative dental materials is

    ⓐ oxyphosphate of zinc

    ⓑ zinc oxide – eugenol

    ⓒ calcium hydroxide

    ⓓ glass ionomer

31. The cement of choice to be placed in a preparation with less than 1 mm of tooth structure over the pulp is

    ⓐ calcium hydroxide

    ⓑ zinc oxide – eugenol

    ⓒ zinc phosphate

    ⓓ glass ionomer

32. Calcium hydroxide formulas used as liners in cavity preparations are available in

① two-paste systems

② premixed systems

③ light-cured systems

④ varnish and powder systems

    ⓐ 1, 2

    ⓑ 2, 3

    ⓒ 1, 2, 3

    ⓓ 2, 4

33. Materials used as varnishes in a cavity preparation are placed

    ⓐ over composite restorations

    ⓑ under composite restorations

    ⓒ before placement of calcium hydroxide

    ⓓ over sterile root canals

34. When preparing tooth enamel or dentin for etching and bonding of composites, the polishing pastes must be

(a) in large particles

(b) in fine particles

(c) mixed with hydrogen peroxide

(d) free of fluorides

(e) mixed with eugenol

35. Zinc phosphate cement is frequently used in restorative dentistry for

(1) temporizing a tooth

(2) insulation in deep preparations

(3) construction of temporary coverage

(4) luting of cast restorations

(a) 1, 3

(b) 2, 4

(c) 1, 2, 3

(d) 4 only

36. Zinc phosphate cement is contraindicated for placement over the pulpal area of a tooth with a deep preparation because it

(a) washes readily under saliva

(b) sets up slowly

(c) is irritating to the pulp

(d) causes pulp resorption

37. Which of the following impression materials may be used to obtain sharp detail of the subgingival margins of a tooth prepared for a cast gold crown?

(1) vinyl polysiloxane

(2) polyether

(3) reversible hydrocolloid

(4) irreversible hydrocolloid

(a) 1, 3

(b) 2, 4

(c) 1, 2, 3

(d) 4 only

38. By law, a dentist must keep a record of

(a) narcotics prescribed

Continued on next page

ⓑ prescription drugs obtained through a telephoned order

ⓒ Schedule III drugs

ⓓ each drug prescribed for or administered to a patient

39. Which of the following are forms of parenteral drug administration?

① sublingual

② rectal

③ subcutaneous

④ intramuscular

⑤ intravenous

ⓐ 1, 2

ⓑ 1, 3

ⓒ 2, 4, 5

ⓓ 3, 4, 5

40. The drugs used to treat allergic reactions are

ⓐ antibodies

ⓑ antihistamines

ⓒ corticosteroids

ⓓ analgesics

41. What is the portion of a written prescription that specifies the name and strength of the drug to be dispensed?

ⓐ R_x

ⓑ heading

ⓒ body

ⓓ closing

42. Which one of the following abbreviations used on a prescription signifies "after meals"?

ⓐ q.i.d.

ⓑ p.r.n.

ⓒ b.i.d.

ⓓ p.c

43. Bacteria in a carious tooth lesion may pass into the pulp by way of the

ⓐ dentinal tubules

ⓑ periapical tissues

(c) lymph system

(d) neutrophils

44. The instrument initially used to enlarge the root canal from which the pulp tissue has been removed is a

    (a) barbed broach

    (b) rat-tail file

    (c) reamer

    (d) spreader

45. Reamer sizes range from

    (a) 10 to 20

    (b) 10 to 40

    (c) 10 to 60

    (d) 10 to 140

46. Which one of the following instruments is NOT placed on the routine endodontic tray for the cleaning and shaping procedure?

    (a) endodontic explorer

    (b) 5- to 6-ml Luer-Lok syringe

    (c) Glick #1

    (d) master apical file

47. Debridement is the process of

    (a) removing existing or potential irritants from the root canal

    (b) flushing debris from the canal space

    (c) gaining access to the pulp chamber

    (d) planing root canal walls before cleaning and shaping

48. The recommended irrigant in root canal debridement is

    (a) distilled water

    (b) carbolic acid

    (c) sodium hypochlorite

    (d) hydrogen peroxide

49. The most commonly used material for root canal obturation is

    (a) silver

    (b) gutta percha

Continued on next page

ⓒ calcium hydroxide

ⓓ zinc oxide – eugenol

50. Most of the sealers used in endodontics are

ⓐ zinc oxides

ⓑ plastics

ⓒ zinc phosphates

ⓓ epoxy cements

51. Sealers should be mixed to a consistency that is

ⓐ dependent on placement technique

ⓑ dependent on type of obturant placed

ⓒ thick

ⓓ thin

52. Disinfection of gutta percha points is achieved by

ⓐ dipping in sodium hypochlorite

ⓑ placing in bead sterilizer

ⓒ dipping in alcohol

ⓓ placing in cold chemical solution

53. A radiograph for accurate measurement of root canal length may be obtained by the use of what technique?

ⓐ long cone

ⓑ short cone

ⓒ parallel

ⓓ bisection of the angle

54. Which of the following is NOT true in regard to the use of hydrogen peroxide for root canal irrigation?

ⓐ it liberates free oxygen

ⓑ to be effective, it should remain in the canal for at least 8 hours

ⓒ if it is not neutralized, it may cause pericementitis

ⓓ it partially disinfects the canal

55. Which one of the following relates to the surgical removal of vital pulp from the tooth?

ⓐ apicoectomy

ⓑ periapical curettage

ⓒ pulpectomy

ⓓ pulpotomy

56. Which of the following is true of chelators?

ⓐ they work quickly

ⓑ they remove canal obstructions to allow passage of instruments

ⓒ they should be placed in a canal only after instrumentation

ⓓ in order to soften dentin, they should be in a canal for several hours

57. The instrument shown below is

ⓐ a rubber base syringe

ⓑ a Luer-Lok syringe

ⓒ an irrigating syringe

ⓓ a root canal gun

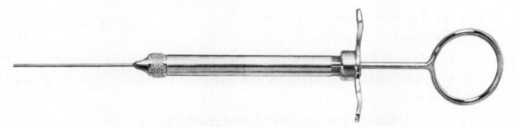

(Courtesy of Union Broach, Division of Moyco Ind., Emigsville, PA.)

58. Percussion is performed on a tooth to determine

ⓐ the mobility of a tooth

ⓑ the sensitivity of a tooth

ⓒ whether or not a fracture is complete

ⓓ whether there is variation in translucency between teeth

59. In what area of the oral cavity is the greatest concentration of hepatitis B virus found?

ⓐ gingival sulcus

ⓑ mucosa

ⓒ dental plaque

ⓓ filiform papillae

60. What is the mandatory first step in inanimate surface asepsis?

    ⓐ application of disinfectant

    ⓑ application of an antiseptic

    ⓒ thorough cleansing of the surface

    ⓓ application of a preparation containing a high concentration of isopro-pyl alcohol

61. Select the answer that most precisely describes the sequence for preparation of instruments for autoclaving

    ① don heavy-gauge rubber gloves

    ② rinse instruments under a hard stream of running water with hinged instruments open

    ③ brush or mechanically clean instruments using a high-pH detergent

    ④ rinse instruments, preferably in distilled water

    ⑤ lubricate all hinged instruments and those with moving parts

        ⓐ 1, 3, 4, 5

        ⓑ 1, 2, 4, 5

        ⓒ 1, 2, 3, 4

        ⓓ 2, 3, 4, 5

62. Before instruments are placed in the sterilizer, bioburden must be reduced because it can

    ① react chemically with instruments and cause them to stain

    ② dry and encrust, thereby protecting microorganisms

    ③ inhibit sterilization

    ④ cause corrosion of instruments, resulting in their dulling

        ⓐ 1, 2

        ⓑ 1, 4

        ⓒ 1, 2, 3

        ⓓ 2, 3, 4

63. Chemicals approved by the Centers for Disease Control (CDC) or American Dental Association for sanitization include

    ① diluted iodophor

    ② alcohol

    ③ sodium hypochlorite

    ④ quarternary ammonium compounds

    ⑤ complex phenol agents

(a) 1, 3
(b) 1, 4
(c) 3, 5
(d) 1, 3, 5
(e) 2, 4, 5

64. Clean-up procedures following dental treatment should be directed to

(1) providing total asepsis on all surfaces
(2) providing rapid action on a wide microbial spectrum
(3) decontaminating items that are potential sources of cross-infection
(4) ensuring that germicides penetrate into equipment crevices

(a) 1, 2, 3
(b) 1, 2, 4
(c) 2, 3, 4
(d) all of the above

65. A comprehensive medical history should be taken for each patient in order to

(1) identify patients with recurrent illnesses
(2) alert practitioners about medical conditions that could be adversely affected by dental treatment
(3) identify medications being taken by patients
(4) identify patients who are infectious disease risks
(5) ascertain the need for enhanced infection control in the office

(a) 1, 2, 3
(b) 1, 4, 5
(c) 2, 3, 4
(d) 3, 4, 5

66. The Occupational Safety and Health Administration (OSHA) states that

(a) clean cotton street wear may be worn when treating dental patients
(b) protective eye ware should be routinely sterilized between patients
(c) fluid-impervious gowns are necessary
(d) clinic attire must NOT be worn while going to or from work

67. Rubber dam use contributes to reducing

(1) pathogen spatter from the operative field
(2) contact of operator's hands with patient's mucosa

Continued on next page

③ the need to follow all steps of the instrument sterilization procedure

④ the need for operators to wear gloves or face mask

(a) 1, 2

(b) 1, 2, 3

(c) 2, 4

(d) all of the above

68. Most exposures to infection that occur among health care providers involve

(a) respiratory pathogen transmission

(b) aerosol spatter

(c) waste disposal

(d) injury from sharps

69. The most acceptable posttreatment of handpieces is

(a) total immersion in a glutaraldehyde solution for 10 minutes

(b) wiping with isopropyl alcohol

(c) exposing to surface disinfectant for 10 minutes

(d) sterilization by steam autoclaving

70. Biologic monitors used to check the achievement of sterilization contain

(a) vegetative bacteria

(b) bacterial spores

(c) attenuated viruses

(d) color-treated paper strips

71. Instruments must be dry before which type of sterilization is undertaken?

(a) dry heat

(b) steam autoclave

(c) glutaraldehyde

(d) chemical vapor

72. Carbon steel instruments must be treated with a corrosion inhibitor before what type of sterilization?

(a) dry heat

(b) steam autoclave

(c) glutaraldehyde

(d) chemical vapor

73. As dictated by universal precautions, surgical gowns, aprons, or laboratory coats that are contacted by body fluids must
    (a) be discarded or laundered after a single use
    (b) not show evidence of having been spotted on a prior contact
    (c) be disposable
    (d) have long sleeves with snug cuff bands

74. Overgloves are used
    (a) when working in the oral cavity
    (b) when performing secondary procedures
    (c) over examination gloves that have been torn or punctured
    (d) over examination gloves that have been contaminated

75. Which of the following gloves may be decontaminated and reused?
    (a) overgloves
    (b) latex (examination) gloves
    (c) utility gloves
    (d) surgical gloves

76. If required to leave the chair, a dental assistant should do which of the following before returning to the patient?
    (a) discard gloves and reglove
    (b) use surgical scrub for cleansing gloved hands
    (c) cover gloved hands with overgloves
    (d) immerse gloved hands in glutaraldehyde solution

77. Which of the following is true in regard to protective masks?
    (a) masks are worn in order to protect patients from infection
    (b) because masks do not come in contact with patients, they may be used for several procedures
    (c) a mask may be placed and removed by any convenient method
    (d) a wet mask is NOT effective

78. Which one of the following is NOT an acceptable form of sterilization?
    (a) autoclaving
    (b) chemical vapor
    (c) boiling water

Continued on next page

(d) dry heat

(e) flash sterilization

79. The consideration that should be given to larger instrument packs wrapped for autoclaving is that they must be

   (a) separated into smaller units before placement

   (b) placed on the bottom of the chamber

   (c) placed at the top of the chamber

   (d) placed at an angle from top to bottom

80. Which of the following surface disinfectants must be freshly mixed each day?

   (a) chlorine dioxide

   (b) iodophors

   (c) synthetic phenol compounds

   (d) sodium hypochlorite

81. Which surface disinfectants produce fumes that are toxic to tissue?

   (a) glutaraldehydes

   (b) iodophors

   (c) synthetic phenol compounds

   (d) sodium hypochlorite

82. How frequently should ultrasonic cleaning solution be changed?

   (a) after processing instruments used on patients considered to be high risk

   (b) when a dipstick test shows it to be of inadequate strength

   (c) daily

   (d) weekly

83. Which one of the following is a suitable instrument wrap for autoclaving?

   (a) snugly wrapped foil

   (b) paper folded envelope style and secured with a safety pin at the flap

   (c) sterilizer bag with end secured by a staple

   (d) muslin wrap secured with tape

84. The type of gloves that should be worn while placing and exposing x-ray films are

   (a) utility gloves

ⓑ overgloves

ⓒ heavy gauge

ⓓ latex

85. After removal from the mouth, an alginate impression should be

    ⓐ sealed in a sterile plastic bag

    ⓑ immersed in disinfectant solution

    ⓒ sprayed with a disinfectant agent

    ⓓ swabbed with 70 percent isopropyl alcohol

86. Failure to equip the dental unit with antiretraction valves can result in

    ⓐ faulty aspiration of oral fluids

    ⓑ difficulty in sterilizing handpiece components

    ⓒ the need to blow out handpiece tubing after each use

    ⓓ water and saliva being drawn into the dental unit fluid line

87. Although gloves are worn for most dental office tasks and procedures, regular antimicrobial hand washing throughout the day is recommended for what reason?

    ⓐ to prevent contamination of gloves when gloving

    ⓑ to protect any open places on the skin

    ⓒ to combat increased skin microbe replication while wearing gloves

    ⓓ to prevent skin allergy to latex gloves

88. Between patients, protective eye wear worn by dental staff should routinely be

    ⓐ chemically sterilized

    ⓑ cleaned

    ⓒ disinfected

    ⓓ wiped with 70 percent alcohol

89. Which of the following infections can be transmitted through the conjunctiva of the eye?

    ⓐ influenza

    ⓑ common cold

    ⓒ hepatitis B

    ⓓ all of the above

    ⓔ none of the above

90. The number of minutes required for topical anesthetic to achieve optimum effectiveness is

    (a) one-half minute

    (b) 1 to 2 minutes

    (c) 2 to 3 minutes

    (d) 3 to 6 minutes

91. To assist in positioning the needle for an infiltration injection, the assistant turns the bevel

    (a) toward the buccal surface

    (b) away from the alveolus

    (c) toward the alveolus

    (d) toward a major vein

92. Anesthetic solution containing epinephrine is recommended for a patient with a heart condition.

    (a) true

    (b) false

93. When passing a loaded syringe to an operator, an assistant

    (a) leaves the needle cap (guard) in place for removal by the operator

    (b) removes the needle cap (guard) immediately after loading the syringe

    (c) removes the needle guard after the syringe is firmly positioned in the operator's hand

    (d) engages the piston rod into the plunger and then removes the needle cap

94. Carpules of local anesthetic solutions containing amber-colored liquid

    (a) are of higher potency

    (b) need to be discarded

    (c) contain epinephrine

    (d) provide longer tissue retention

95. When an assistant passes a local anesthetic syringe into the operator's hand, the

    (1) syringe is laid in the operator's open palm

    (2) ring end of the syringe is passed first

    (3) ring is fitted onto the operator's thumb

    (4) needle cover is removed from the syringe before passing

(a) 1, 3
(b) 1, 4
(c) 1, 2, 3
(d) 3, 4

96. Which of the following first aid measures is recommended when an accidental needle stick has occurred?

① squeeze the wound until it bleeds
② cleanse the wound by holding it under running water
③ disinfect the site with iodophor or a bleach solution
④ seek antibiotic treatment

(a) 1, 3
(b) 2 only
(c) 1, 2, 3
(d) 4 only

97. In addition to topical ointment and a cotton swab, the setup prepared for regional anesthesia of the mandibular inferior alveolar nerve includes

(a) gauze square and anesthetic Carpule
(b) gauze square and syringe with a long needle
(c) gauze square and syringe with a short needle
(d) syringe with either a short or long needle

98. When assisting an oral surgeon with a patient under Stage 3 general anesthesia, which of the following are essential

① placement of throat packs to prevent aspiration of a foreign object
② constant monitoring of the size of the patient's pupils
③ maintenance of the patient's airway
④ frequent aspiration of the trachea and soft palate

(a) 1, 2
(b) 1, 3
(c) 1, 2, 3
(d) 2, 3, 4

99. A candidate for oral surgery under general anesthesia is strongly advised to

(a) see a physician for a physical examination just before the appointment
(b) avoid eating for 6 to 8 hours before the appointment

Continued on next page

ⓒ take mega doses of vitamin E for a week prior to the appointment

ⓓ take aspirin before the appointment

100. Which of the following are true of the herpes simplex virus?

① it is a disease of young adults

② it may be dormant for a period of years

③ its sores always develop at the same place

④ it may be transmitted through saliva

ⓐ 1, 2

ⓑ 1, 3

ⓒ 1, 4

ⓓ 2, 3

ⓔ 2, 3, 4

101. Pellegra, cheilosis, some forms of glossitis, and some forms of anemia are caused by a deficiency of what vitamin?

ⓐ B complex

ⓑ C

ⓒ E

ⓓ A

102. A biopsy is mandatory to establish a definitive diagnosis of which of the following conditions

ⓐ leukoedema

ⓑ leukoplakia

ⓒ follicular keratosis

ⓓ lichen planus

103. Cells responsible for immune responses are organized into what body system?

ⓐ alimentary

ⓑ cardiovascular

ⓒ circulatory

ⓓ lymphatic

104. Which of the following are symptoms of hyperglycemia?

① clammy skin

② vertigo

③ acetone breath
④ rapid weak pulse
⑤ dry mouth
  ⓐ 1, 2, 3
  ⓑ 1, 3, 4
  ⓒ 2, 3, 5
  ⓓ 3, 4, 5

105. The form of bacteria most resistant to destruction is
  ⓐ rod shaped
  ⓑ capsulated
  ⓒ spore
  ⓓ spiral shaped with flexible walls

106. Infectious agents that are able to replicate only in living cells are
  ⓐ bacterial spores
  ⓑ viruses
  ⓒ protozoa
  ⓓ bacterial capsules

107. Immunity is dependent on the presence of
  ⓐ allergens
  ⓑ antigens
  ⓒ abnormalities
  ⓓ antibodies

108. Which of the following are agents to promote the clotting of blood?
  ① vitamin A
  ② epinephrine
  ③ thrombin
  ④ tannic acid
  ⓐ 1, 2
  ⓑ 1, 2, 3
  ⓒ 2, 3, 4
  ⓓ 3, 4

109. Myocardial infarction occurs when

    (a) there is ventricular standstill

    (b) one or more coronary arteries become blocked

    (c) ventricular fibrillation occurs

    (d) spasms occur in the heart muscle

110. If during cardiopulmonary resuscitation (CPR) a patient's pupils are dilated when exposed to light, the rescuer knows that

    (a) an insufficient amount of oxygenated blood is reaching the brain

    (b) the patient is a drug abuser

    (c) the patient will soon return to consciousness

    (d) the head is not properly tilted

111. Which of the following drugs should be administered intravenously for hypoglycemic coma?

    (a) dextrose 50 percent

    (b) dextrose 5 percent

    (c) Benadryl

    (d) atropine

112. Which one of the following is a necessary procedure when an Ambu bag is in use?

    (a) the mask is placed over the patient's mouth only

    (b) head tilt is maintained

    (c) the bag is squeezed once every 12 seconds when working on an adult

    (d) the patient is not allowed to exhale and so deflate the bag

113. Normally during the Heimlich maneuver, patients are

    (a) placed in the supine position

    (b) instructed to close their mouth

    (c) told to tilt their head back

    (d) directed to keep the mouth open

114. A conscious patient with a blocked airway may be

    (a) given the abdominal thrust

    (b) given a large glass of water

    (c) positioned in a supine position

    (d) delivered a forceful blow in the upper back

115. If a patient is suffering a myocardial infarction, the first aid procedure should include

   ① placing the patient in a supine position

   ② calling 911 (paramedics)

   ③ administering 100 percent oxygen

   ④ keeping the patient quiet

      ⓐ 1, 3

      ⓑ 2, 4

      ⓒ 2, 3, 4

      ⓓ all of the above

116. If a patient in pulmonary arrest has ceased breathing, emergency first aid should include

   ① calling 911

   ② placing the patient in a supine position

   ③ checking for a foreign object in the airway

   ④ maintaining the airway

   ⑤ checking for breathing and pulse

      ⓐ 1, 2, 3

      ⓑ 1, 2, 3, 4

      ⓒ 2, 4, 5

      ⓓ all of the above

117. Which of the following are acceptable methods for administering artificial ventilation?

      ⓐ abdominal thrust

      ⓑ mouth-to-mouth

      ⓒ mouth-to-nose

      ⓓ artificial airway

      ⓔ a, b, c

118. The sequence in which a two-rescuer team delivers CPR to an unconscious nonbreathing patient is

      ⓐ 1 breath/artificial ventilation to 2 chest impressions

      ⓑ 1 breath/artificial ventilation to 5 chest impressions

      ⓒ 2 breaths/artificial ventilations to 5 chest impressions

      ⓓ 2 breaths/artificial ventilations to 15 chest impressions

119. Administering CPR to an infant or a small child requires which changes from the adult CPR method?

    ① reducing pressure on the chest
    ② increasing pressure on the chest
    ③ reducing the force of artificial ventilation
    ④ increasing the force of artificial ventilation

        ⓐ 1, 2
        ⓑ 1, 3
        ⓒ 2, 3
        ⓓ 2, 4

120. Confinement in an airtight container and placement in a boiling water bath is the first step in preparation of which of the following impression materials?

        ⓐ irreversible hydrocolloid
        ⓑ polysulfide elastomer
        ⓒ reversible hydrocolloid
        ⓓ polyether elastomer

121. In the business office, accounts payable are

        ⓐ fees owed by patients
        ⓑ accounts paid by patients
        ⓒ monies owed by the dental practice
        ⓓ monies disbursed by the dental practice

122. Fixed overhead includes

        ⓐ all salaries
        ⓑ rent
        ⓒ laboratory fees
        ⓓ supplies
        ⓔ a, b
        ⓕ b, c, d

123. To provide adequate space for the impression material when constructing a custom impression tray, the cast is covered with

        ⓐ tinfoil
        ⓑ two layers of base plate wax
        ⓒ tray adhesive
        ⓓ tray compound

124. Vinyl polysiloxane impression material is supplied in several forms including
    ① light bodied
    ② regular bodied
    ③ heavy bodied
    ④ liquid
    ⑤ gel
        ⓐ 1, 2, 3
        ⓑ 1, 3, 4
        ⓒ 1, 3, 5
        ⓓ all of the above

125. Polysulfide, vinyl polysiloxane, and polyether impression materials are composed of a
        ⓐ retarder
        ⓑ base
        ⓒ catalyst
        ⓓ a, c
        ⓔ b, c

126. The main advantage to the use of reversible hydrocolloid impression material is that it provides
        ⓐ sharp detail of the prepared teeth
        ⓑ elasticity when removed from deep undercuts
        ⓒ long curing time on the laboratory bench
        ⓓ distortion only after prolonged exposure to air

127. Which of the following provides "stops" within a custom tray?
        ⓐ several layers of base plate wax placed on the cast
        ⓑ two coatings of tray adhesive placed on the cast
        ⓒ three to four small holes cut into the base plate wax
        ⓓ a ridge of base plate wax at the posterior dimension

128. A dental product that is back ordered is one that
        ⓐ is currently unavailable for delivery
        ⓑ has a short shelf life
        ⓒ is needed immediately
        ⓓ requires a requisition

129. Expendable items include

   ① extraction forceps

   ② gutta percha points

   ③ film mounts

   ④ rubber dam clamps

     ⓐ 1, 2

     ⓑ 2, 3

     ⓒ 2, 4

     ⓓ all of the above

130. When writing a check, information that is NOT recorded in the check register is the

     ⓐ name of the payee

     ⓑ amount of the check

     ⓒ name of the payor

     ⓓ number of the check

131. Canceled checks are those that

     ⓐ have been charged against the checking account

     ⓑ have been written

     ⓒ have been voided because of an error

     ⓓ create an overdraft

132. If $50.00 is the amount of money kept in petty cash, a $29.00 check is written for the purchase of stamps, and $16.83 in cash is spent on miscellaneous items, the amount necessary to replenish the petty cash fund is

     ⓐ $16.83

     ⓑ $29.00

     ⓒ $33.17

     ⓓ $45.83

133. W-4 forms must be completed by an employee

     ⓐ at the beginning of employment

     ⓑ at the end of each quarter

     ⓒ when leaving a position of employment

     ⓓ only when he or she has dependents

134. A report of all taxable wages paid to each employee must be filed once each:

    (a) year

    (b) month

    (c) quarter

    (d) 6-month period

135. A raised check is one that

    (a) is nonnegotiable

    (b) has extra dollars added

    (c) has been returned because of insufficient funds

    (d) had insufficient funds but clears the bank when redeposited

136. In handling silver amalgam for a restoration, it is important to

    (a) triturate according to the manufacturer's recommendation

    (b) prevent contamination

    (c) place, condense, and carve while the mass is pliable

    (d) polish while margins are pliable

    (e) a, b, c

    (f) a, c, d

137. Which of the following matrices may be used for placement of a Class II two-surface amalgam restoration on a primary tooth?

    (1) T band

    (2) Tofflemire band

    (3) metal strip

    (4) Mylar strip

        (a) 1, 3

        (b) 2, 4

        (c) 1, 2, 3

        (d) 4 only

138. The criteria for an acceptable matrix for an amalgam restoration are that it be

    (1) easy to apply

    (2) transparent

    (3) rigid

    (4) flexible

        (a) 1, 2

        (b) 1, 3

Continued on next page

    (c) 1, 4

    (d) 2, 4

139. Which tooth surface is NOT covered by a posterior three-quarter crown?

    (a) lingual

    (b) occlusal

    (c) facial

    (d) mesial or distal

140. Units of a bridge are known as

    (a) pontics

    (b) abutments

    (c) joints

    (d) a, b

    (e) all of the above

141. The number of retention pins normally placed in a mandibular second molar is

    (a) 5

    (b) 4

    (c) 3

    (d) 2

142. The number of retention pins normally placed on a maxillary cuspid is

    (a) 4

    (b) 3

    (c) 2

    (d) 1

143. Materials used for crown core build-up include

    (1) zinc oxide–eugenol

    (2) calcium hydroxide

    (3) amalgam

    (4) reinforced glass ionomer

    (5) composite

        (a) 1, 2, 3

        (b) 1, 3, 5

(c) 2, 3, 4

(d) 3, 4, 5

144. The use of retraction cord impregnated with racemic epinephrine is contraindicated for patients suffering from

(a) diabetes

(b) cardiovascular disease

(c) epileptic seizures

(d) osteoporosis

145. Retraction cord is normally left in place for how many minutes?

(a) 2 to 4

(b) 5 to 7

(c) 10 to 12

(d) 25 to 30

146. Retraction cord is packed with a blunt instrument

(a) from lingual to facial

(b) from mesial to distal

(c) in a clockwise direction

(d) in a counterclockwise direction

147. Stops are formed in a custom tray to

(a) ensure correct mesial/distal placement of tray

(b) prevent occlusal stress

(c) allow adequate space for impression material

(d) provide retention for impression material

148. When seated, a temporary aluminum crown should extend beyond the gingival margin of the prepared tooth no farther than

(a) 1.0 mm

(b) 0.5 mm

(c) 0.3 mm

(d) 0.2 mm

149. In what area of a wax pattern is a sprue placed?

(a) on the occlusal or incisal surfaces

Continued on next page

ⓑ on the smoothest area

ⓒ toward the gingival margin

ⓓ on the heaviest area

150. The flange of a mandibular denture extends over the genial tubercles, which are located

ⓐ lingual to the centrals

ⓑ lingual to the canines

ⓒ distal to the last molars

ⓓ facial to the centrals

151. Post damming is provided in the area of the

ⓐ oblique ridge

ⓑ transverse palatine suture

ⓒ buccinator crest

ⓓ greater palatine foramen

152. The usual reason for relining an immediate denture a few months after delivery is

ⓐ slow healing of surgical area

ⓑ a need to reconstruct a post dam

ⓒ bite closure

ⓓ alveolar ridge resorption

153. Dental plaque may be described to patients as

① an essential coating of the cervical areas of the teeth

② a soft thin film of food debris, dead epithelial cells, and mucin

③ an antagonist to calculus formation

④ an etiologic agent in the development of caries and periodontal disease

ⓐ 1, 2

ⓑ 2, 3

ⓒ 2, 4

ⓓ 3, 4

154. Which of the following statements are true in regard to plaque control?

ⓐ the Bass brushing technique is always preferred

ⓑ oral irrigation should be used for removal of stainable plaque

(c) step-by-step control procedures should be learned by all patients

(d) conscientious home care helps prevents plaque, stain, and calculus

155. Chronic gingivitis is always caused by

(a) local irritants

(b) systemic conditions

(c) poor nutrition

(d) calculus

156. An explanation to patients in regard to the need for a periodontal pack after surgery should include which of the following?

(1) it prevents postoperative discomfort

(2) it prevents later development of periodontal pockets

(3) it aids healing

(4) it helps to retain mobile teeth

(a) 1, 2

(b) 1, 2, 3

(c) 1, 3, 4

(d) 3, 4

157. Which of the following postsurgical instructions are correct?

(1) rinse immediately on arriving at home

(2) immediately resume all daily activities

(3) increase intake of water and fruit juices

(4) call the dental office if swelling is sustained or painful

(5) report to the office immediately if any bleeding occurs

(a) 1, 2, 3

(b) 2, 3, 4

(c) 3, 4

(d) 4, 5

158. After periodontal pack removal, patients are instructed to immediately begin a plaque control program that includes

(1) vigorous brushing

(2) the use of dental floss or dental tape

(3) irrigation by water

(4) interdental massage with toothpicks

Continued on next page

ⓐ 1, 2, 3
ⓑ 2, 3
ⓒ 3, 4
ⓓ 4, 5

159. What grasp is used for the prophy angle during coronal polish?

ⓐ pen
ⓑ modified pen
ⓒ palm
ⓓ palm thrust

160. The agent that is usually used to remove stains on proximal surfaces of anterior teeth is

ⓐ dental tape with an abrasive
ⓑ dental floss with an abrasive
ⓒ dental floss or tape without an abrasive
ⓓ polishing strip

161. Bristle brushes are usually used on what tooth areas?

ⓐ cervical third
ⓑ in the presence of metal fillings
ⓒ occlusal surfaces
ⓓ gingival third of the lingual surface

162. Which one of the following is NOT a goal in periodontal instrument sharpening?

ⓐ preserve the burnishing effect of the instrument
ⓑ increase instrument working efficiency
ⓒ preserve the shape and proportional dimensions
ⓓ maintain and restore knifelike cutting edges

163. Which one of the following is NOT included in the tray setup for coronal polishing?

ⓐ porte polisher
ⓑ high-velocity evacuation tip
ⓒ plastic floss threader
ⓓ high-speed handpiece

164. Which of the following terms best describes a sharply defined wedge-shaped depression in the cervical area of the facial surface of a tooth?

    (a) abrasion

    (b) attrition

    (c) distortion

    (d) erosion

165. Tinted sealants are advocated instead of transparent sealants because they

    (a) demonstrate superior retention rates

    (b) are more effective in caries prevention

    (c) may be more easily monitored in regard to retention

    (d) demonstrate more uniform setting qualities

166. The instrument used to remove the sharp edges of the alveolar crest after extraction is a

    (a) forceps

    (b) curette

    (c) rongeur

    (d) bone chisel

167. Cold packs used to control swelling should

    (a) be placed during the first 24 hours after surgery

    (b) be used intermittently with heat packs

    (c) remain on the involved area for at least 8 hours

    (d) NOT be placed in the presence of pain

168. What occurs if a blood clot does not remain in the socket after an extraction?

    (a) granulation tissue is produced

    (b) a gram-positive infection develops

    (c) severe bleeding may be expected

    (d) the bone is exposed

169. The type of suture that is absorbed by the body is

    (a) nylon

    (b) silk

    (c) cotton

    (d) gut

170. Oral surgery procedures demand that the aseptic technique begin with

    (a) hand scrubbing

    (b) preparation of the patient

    (c) preliminary arrangement of the operatory

    (d) application of gloves by the operator

171. Which one of the following is used to elevate an impacted tooth or a tooth with a broken crown from its socket?

    (a) exolever

    (b) apical elevator

    (c) periosteal elevator

    (d) T-handle root elevator

172. Which of the following are the least cariogenic snack foods?

    (a) candy bars, jelly beans, caramel corn

    (b) doughnuts, raisins, chocolate milk

    (c) peanuts, pretzels, popcorn

    (d) apple, cheese, breath mints

173. Which of the following groups of snack foods would NOT be advised because they contribute the fewest essential nutrients to the diet?

    (a) milk and cheese

    (b) nuts and hard boiled eggs

    (c) sugar-free gelatins and soft drinks

    (d) celery and carrot sticks

174. Which nutrients serve as major sources of energy for most people?

    (a) complex carbohydrates

    (b) proteins

    (c) fats

    (d) vitamin supplements

175. Which nutrients serve as the fundamental structural element of every cell?

    (a) carbohydrates

    (b) proteins

    (c) fats

    (d) complex carbohydrates

176. For resuscitative procedures in a dental office, the most effective agent is

    (a) nitrous oxide

    (b) epinephrine

    (c) Demerol

    (d) oxygen

177. To alleviate apprehension and fear pending treatment, a dentist may administer nitrous oxide and oxygen to produce a state of

    (a) anesthesia

    (b) amnesia

    (c) relative analgesia

    (d) excitement

178. Relative analgesia is contraindicated

    (a) in patients with respiratory problems

    (b) when it is difficult to communicate with the patient

    (c) in patients older than 60 years

    (d) in apprehensive patients

    (e) a, b

179. What is the role of the assistant when assisting with the administration of nitrous oxide and oxygen?

    (1) assist in the administration of these gases via the intravenous route

    (2) function under the direct supervision of the dentist

    (3) assist with the administration of these agents to alleviate respiratory problems

    (4) constantly monitor the tanks

    (5) start the flow of nitrous oxide and oxygen at the patient's baseline

        (a) 1, 3

        (b) 2, 4

        (c) 2, 4, 5

        (d) 3, 5

180. After baseline values are achieved when administering nitrous oxide and oxygen to a patient,

    (a) the assistant adjusts the levels of the gases

    (b) the dentist closes the vent valve

    (c) the patient maintains the level of gases

    (d) the dental team continues to monitor the patient and the equipment

181. When a patient is *fully alert* after administration of nitrous oxide and oxygen

① the mask is removed

② the chair back is slowly raised upright

③ the baseline is recorded on the patient's chart

④ oxygen is administered for a minimum of 1 minute

    ⓐ 1, 2

    ⓑ 2, 3

    ⓒ 1, 2, 3

    ⓓ 2, 4

182. To prevent needle-stick injury

    ⓐ the guard should immediately be placed over the end of the used needle

    ⓑ the used needle should immediately be removed and placed in a sharps container

    ⓒ the used needle should be placed into the open end of a guard before its removal from the syringe

    ⓓ the used needle should be dipped into iodophor disinfecting solution before removal from the syringe

183. Reversible impression materials are used in construction of which of the following?

① temporary coverage

② complete dentures

③ custom trays

④ implants

⑤ study casts

    ⓐ 1, 2, 3

    ⓑ 1, 3, 4

    ⓒ 2, 4

    ⓓ 2, 4, 5

184. Irreversible hydrocolloid impression materials used in construction of opposing arch casts and study casts are referred to as

① elastomers

② silicone carbides

③ polycarboxylates

④ alginates

    ⓐ 1, 3

    ⓑ 2, 4

ⓒ 2, 3, 4

ⓓ 4 only

185. A bite registration of a patient's occlusion is obtained by using

① alginate material

② zinc oxide impression pastes

③ impression compound

④ vinyl polysiloxane material

ⓐ 1, 3

ⓑ 1, 2, 3

ⓒ 2, 4

ⓓ 4 only

186. Type II gypsum material is referred to as

ⓐ die stone

ⓑ impression plaster

ⓒ model plaster

ⓓ dental stone

187. Type IV gypsum material is referred to as

① high-strength dental stone

② densite

③ improved dental stone

④ laboratory plaster

ⓐ 1, 3

ⓑ 1, 2, 3

ⓒ 2, 4

ⓓ 4 only

188. When mixing gypsum material for a Type IV stone cast, the amount of water added to 100 grams of powder should be

ⓐ 22 ml

ⓑ 30 ml

ⓒ 40 to 50 ml

ⓓ 50 to 60 ml

189. Silver amalgam is a fusion of

① silver

② titanium

③ copper

④ platinum

⑤ mercury

ⓐ 1, 2, 3

ⓑ 1, 3, 4

ⓒ 1, 2, 3, 5

ⓓ 3, 4, 5

190. The disadvantages of silver amalgam are that it

① has a high rate of thermal conductivity

② fails to bond to tooth structure

③ has a tendency to tarnish if not polished

④ is difficult to manipulate

ⓐ 1, 3

ⓑ 2, 4

ⓒ 1, 2, 3

ⓓ 1, 3, 4

191. Silver amalgam is precapsulated, covered and triturated in an amalgamator, and dispensed into the cavity preparation by means of an amalgam carrier in order to

ⓐ prevent oxidation of the alloy

ⓑ reduce exposure of the dental team to mercury vapors

ⓒ reduce shrinkage of the finished restoration

ⓓ prevent discoloration of the amalgam

192. The synthetic resins frequently used for temporary coverage repairs are

ⓐ self-polymerizing

ⓑ heat cured

ⓒ white light cured

ⓓ microfilled composites

193. Which of the following may be used to accomplish rubber dam ligation?

ⓐ dental floss placed at the proximal surface of the tooth opposite the anchor tooth

ⓑ inversion of dam margins into the gingival sulcus

ⓒ knotted dental floss passed through interproximal contacts

ⓓ dental floss placed at the interproximal space mesial to the anchor tooth

194. Which of the following is used to keep the margins of a rubber dam away from the face?

ⓐ ligation

ⓑ frame

ⓒ clamp

ⓓ beaver-tail burnisher

195. Which of the following apply when placing a rubber dam over a three-unit fixed bridge?

① the anchor tooth punch hole is larger

② the anchor tooth punch hole is smaller

③ facial and lingual punch holes are made toward the unclamped abutment

④ abutment teeth are covered

ⓐ 1, 3

ⓑ 2, 3

ⓒ 2, 4

ⓓ 4 only

196. After the frame, clamp, ligation, and dam are removed, a used rubber dam is checked for

① missing fragments

② tears

③ cut septa

④ blood

ⓐ 1, 2

ⓑ 2, 3

ⓒ 1, 2, 3

ⓓ 2, 3, 4

197. Zinc phosphate cement is frequently used

① in temporizing a tooth

② as an insulation base

③ in constructing temporary coverage

④ in luting of cast restorations

Continued on next page

      ⓐ 1, 3

      ⓑ 1, 2, 3

      ⓒ 2, 4

      ⓓ 4 only

198. Zinc phosphate cement is indicated for luting because it

      ⓐ readily bonds with tooth dentin

      ⓑ does not break down in the presence of saliva

      ⓒ provides long lasting adherence when margins are protected

      ⓓ is of a strength comparable to enamel

199. Zinc phosphate cement is placed over calcium hydroxide to serve as

      ⓐ an insulating base

      ⓑ a temporizing agent

      ⓒ a luting agent

      ⓓ a palliative agent

200. Instrumentation for mixing zinc phosphate cement includes

      ① a cool, dry glass slab

      ② a rigid steel spatula

      ③ dispensers for the powder and liquid

      ④ a waxed paper pad

      ⑤ a bone spatula

          ⓐ 1, 2

          ⓑ 1, 3

          ⓒ 2, 3, 4

          ⓓ 3, 4, 5

201. One criterion for zinc phosphate cement mix used for cementation is that it must

      ⓐ hang in a drop 1/2 inch from the spatula

      ⓑ set in 90 seconds

      ⓒ set in 60 seconds

      ⓓ hang in a drop 1 inch from the spatula

202. To retard the setting of zinc phosphate cement used for cementation, an assistant

ⓐ uses equal portions of powder and liquid and lets the mix stand for 15 seconds

ⓑ incorporates a very small amount of powder into the liquid and lets the mix stand for 15 seconds

ⓒ incorporates all the powder into the liquid and spatulates rapidly

ⓓ uses twice as much liquid as powder and spatulates rapidly

203. Zinc oxide–eugenol cement is effective when used as

① a temporary restoration (short term)

② a palliative agent

③ an insulating base over calcium hydroxide

④ a permanent cementing agent

    ⓐ 1, 3

    ⓑ 1, 2, 3

    ⓒ 2, 4

    ⓓ 2, 3, 4

204. Zinc oxide–eugenol cement used for temporary coverage should

① be of medium viscosity

② flow freely

③ set within 5 minutes

④ be of puttylike viscosity

    ⓐ 1, 2

    ⓑ 1, 4

    ⓒ 1, 2, 3

    ⓓ 2, 3, 4

205. The most effective chemotherapeutic method of caries control is

    ⓐ tooth brushing

    ⓑ regular coronal polishing

    ⓒ the use of fluoride

    ⓓ the use of plaque retardants

206. Which of the following materials would be placed to restore a Class IV fracture?

① zinc oxide–eugenol base

② calcium hydroxide

③ silver amalgam

④ microfilled composite

Continued on next page

(a) 1, 3
(b) 1, 4
(c) 2, 3
(d) 2, 4

207. In the instrument formula 10-7-14, the 7 refers to the

(a) angle formed by the handle and the blade
(b) length of the blade
(c) width of the blade
(d) angle formed by the cutting edge and the handle

208. When seating a rubber dam clamp, the procedure is to

(a) place the facial jaws first
(b) place the lingual jaws first
(c) tip the forceps to the lingual and seat both jaws at the same time
(d) achieve jaw placement depending on the integrity of the cusps

209. An instrument of choice for rubber dam inversion is the

(a) ball burnisher
(b) cleoid
(c) binangle chisel
(d) beaver-tail burnisher

210. When using the reverse pen grasp while checking on a maxillary central incisor, the fulcrum is on the

(a) maxillary cuspid
(b) maxillary premolar area
(c) mandibular teeth
(d) chin

211. The correct handpiece grasp when operating on the occlusal surface of a mandibular left first molar uses which digits?

(a) thumb, forefinger, and side of the middle finger
(b) thumb, forefinger, and end of the middle finger
(c) thumb, forefinger, and end of the middle finger with the ring finger on the handpiece
(d) thumb, forefinger, and end of middle finger with the ring finger based on mandibular anteriors

212. Abrasive agents are used to polish

① enamel

② plastic fillings

③ amalgam fillings

④ unfilled resin glazes

ⓐ 1 only

ⓑ 3 only

ⓒ 2, 3

ⓓ 3, 4

213. Which of the following are true of dental hoes?

① they are used in a scraping manner

② they are used for the removal of carious dentin

③ they are always beveled on the back side

④ they may be contra-angled

ⓐ 1, 2

ⓑ 1, 3

ⓒ 1, 3, 4

ⓓ 2, 3, 4

214. When using a pen grasp while working on the mandible, which finger acts as a fulcrum against the teeth?

ⓐ index finger

ⓑ little finger

ⓒ ring finger

ⓓ middle finger

215. Which is true in regard to rubber dam lubricants?

ⓐ they are placed on the facial side of the dam

ⓑ soap is an excellent lubricant

ⓒ oil-soluble lubricants are preferable to water-soluble ones

ⓓ a rubber dam cannot be applied without a lubricant

216. An anterior rubber dam application for operative purposes should include what minimum number of teeth?

ⓐ 10

ⓑ 8

Continued on next page

ⓒ 7

ⓓ 3

217. After the rubber dam has been placed over the clamped tooth, the operator next

ⓐ stretches the dam over the tooth anterior to it

ⓑ places a rubber dam napkin

ⓒ stretches the dam over the opposite tooth

ⓓ forces the dam over all the teeth involved

218. A #212 clamp is usually used for isolation of which classification of cavity?

ⓐ II

ⓑ III

ⓒ IV

ⓓ V

ⓔ VI

219. When using a Tofflemire retainer, the inner nut is turned clockwise to

ⓐ make the loop smaller

ⓑ enlarge the loop

ⓒ adjust the diagonal slot

ⓓ guide the loop through the appropriate channel

ⓔ tighten the spindle

220. When practicing four-handed dentistry, the assistant should be positioned

ⓐ even with the operator

ⓑ 4 to 6 inches lower than the operator

ⓒ 4 to 6 inches above the operator

ⓓ directly across from the operator

221. In what position should the operator be when working on the lingual surface of a patient's anterior teeth?

ⓐ 12 o'clock

ⓑ 11 o'clock

ⓒ 9 o'clock

ⓓ 7 to 9 o'clock

222. When an anesthetic syringe is passed to the operator, the bevel of the needle should be toward

(a) the patient

(b) the operator

(c) the tooth to be anesthetized

(d) the bone at the injection site

223. The instrument transfer zone is that area

(a) adjacent to the oral cavity

(b) at the side of the patient's head

(c) below the patient's chin

(d) across the patient's lap

224. Which of the following instruments may be used for carving anatomic detail in restorations?

(1) file

(2) Tanner carver

(3) Hollenback carver

(4) burnisher

(5) Wedelstaedt chisel

    (a) 1, 2, 3

    (b) 1, 4, 5

    (c) 2, 3, 4

    (d) 2, 4, 5

225. The most versatile hand grasp for high-velocity evacuations is the

(a) pen

(b) overhand

(c) palm

(d) reverse pen

226. A rubber dam is NOT removed until

(a) the matrix and wedge have been removed

(b) preliminary carving of the occlusal surface has been completed

(c) final occlusal adjustments are necessary

(d) the final polish has been completed

227. The two most commonly used rubber dam frames are the

(1) Ferrier

Continued on next page

②　Woodbury

③　Glidden

④　Young

⑤　anterior

    ⓐ 1, 2

    ⓑ 2, 3

    ⓒ 2, 4

    ⓓ 3, 5

228. Which of the following types of composite resins may produce a smooth surface when cured and polished?

    ⓐ quartz-filled resin

    ⓑ microfilled resin

    ⓒ macrofilled resin

    ⓓ silica-filled resin

229. When applying a gel-type etchant, the gel is left in contact with the enamel approximately

    ⓐ 15 seconds

    ⓑ 30 seconds

    ⓒ 45 seconds

    ⓓ 60 seconds

230. After pit and fissure sealants are applied to tooth enamel, patients should be scheduled for a checkup in

    ⓐ 3 months

    ⓑ 6 months

    ⓒ 1 year

    ⓓ 2 years

231. Composite resins may adapt to which of the following?

①　cast gold restorations

②　bonded enamel veneers

③　silver amalgam

    ⓐ 1 only

    ⓑ 3 only

    ⓒ 1, 2

    ⓓ 1, 2, 3

232. Properly etched tooth enamel when rinsed and dried appears
   ⓐ frosty, whitish
   ⓑ glossy
   ⓒ dark, frosty
   ⓓ streaked, gray

233. How long should a curing light be applied to each tooth during the curing of enamel sealants?
   ⓐ 1 to 2 seconds
   ⓑ 3 to 4 seconds
   ⓒ 5 to 10 seconds
   ⓓ 10 to 20 seconds

234. Preparation of the teeth for treatment with pit and fissure sealants includes the use of
   ① a soft prophy brush
   ② soft rubber prophy cups
   ③ fluoride abrasive
   ④ fluoride-free abrasive
   ⑤ a #10 round bur
   ⓐ 1, 3
   ⓑ 1, 4, 5
   ⓒ 2, 4
   ⓓ 2, 4, 5

235. When preparing the teeth for pit and fissure sealants, which step follows rinsing and drying the polished teeth?
   ⓐ applying etching liquid or gel
   ⓑ applying the sealant material
   ⓒ light curing the etching liquid
   ⓓ light curing the sealant material

236. The teeth most frequently moved by extraoral anchorage are the
   ⓐ maxillary cuspids
   ⓑ mandibular premolars
   ⓒ maxillary molars
   ⓓ maxillary premolars

237. Anchorage in which all resistance units are confined to one arch is

    (a) simple arch

    (b) reciprocal

    (c) intermandibular

    (d) intramaxillary

238. Brackets are bonded with which of the following materials?

    (a) zinc phosphate

    (b) calcium hydroxide

    (c) glass ionomer

    (d) composite resin

239. Bonded brackets are removed using which instrument?

    (a) pin and ligature cutter

    (b) bird beak pliers

    (c) How pliers

    (d) Schure instrument

240. In regard to the removal of steel spring separators,

    (a) the instrument of choice for removal is a Schure scaler

    (b) the helix is engaged and lifted upward

    (c) removal is from the lingual aspect

    (d) the upper arm is disengaged from the lingual embrasure using long beak pliers

241. Orthodontic bands with buccal tubes are seated on which teeth?

    (a) canines

    (b) premolars

    (c) first molars

    (d) most posterior molars

242. The instrument of choice for measuring the height of placement of anterior orthodontic bands is a

    (a) millimeter ruler

    (b) Boley gauge

    (c) Venier scale

    (d) Boone gauge

243. Which of the following can be caused by a tongue thrust habit?

    (a) closed bite

    (b) cross-bite

    (c) diastema

    (d) open bite

244. The preservation of arch length is the function of

    (a) a Crozat appliance

    (b) an Andresen appliance

    (c) a cantilevered crown

    (d) a space maintainer

245. The recommended grasp of ligature tying pliers is the

    (a) pen

    (b) reverse pen

    (c) palm thrust

    (d) palm thumb

246. Soldered attachments on a maxillary molar band may include

    (1) an arch wire tube

    (2) a facial bracket

    (3) a head gear tube

    (4) a lingual cleat

        (a) 1, 2, 3

        (b) 1, 2, 4

        (c) 1, 3, 4

        (d) 2, 3, 4

247. Which of the following instruments may be used for removing bands?

    (1) band removal pliers

    (2) Schure instrument

    (3) heavy scaler

    (4) How pliers

        (a) 1 only

        (b) 1, 2, 3

        (c) 1, 2, 4

        (d) 2, 3, 4

248. During a coronal polishing procedure, the occlusal surfaces of the posterior teeth are cleaned with a

(a) rubber cup and abrasive

(b) porte polisher

(c) soft-bristled brush and abrasive

(d) red stone and mild abrasive

249. For safety and control during a coronal polishing, the hand holding the right-angle handpiece is positioned on the

(1) incisal edge of the anteriors

(2) occlusal surface of the posteriors

(3) facial surface of the teeth

(4) teeth in the same quadrant to be polished

(a) 1, 3

(b) 2, 4

(c) 3, 4

(d) 1, 2, 4

250. During a coronal polishing procedure, the hand holding and directing the right-angle handpiece is stabilized by

(a) thumb hooked under the chin

(b) the use of bent cotton rolls

(c) the base of the hand

(d) means of a fulcrum

251. A coronal polishing procedure

(a) covers beyond the anatomic crown of the tooth

(b) covers beyond the clinical crown of the tooth

(c) is done with a lifting, sweeping, and stroking motion

(d) is done with the polishing cup directed toward the gingiva

252. The intent of a coronal polishing procedure is to remove

(1) plaque

(2) intrinsic stains

(3) extrinsic stains

(4) calculus

(5) enamel mottling

(a) 1, 2
(b) 1, 3
(c) 3, 4
(d) 3, 4, 5

253. When choosing abrasive material for a coronal polishing procedure, it is important to select

(a) the finest particle size
(b) the least abrasive action
(c) one that will make a slurry when mixed with water
(d) one that will make a slurry when mixed with a fluoride base

254. A pulpectomy refers to

(a) a vital pulpotomy
(b) direct pulp capping
(c) total removal of the coronal pulp
(d) total removal of the pulp in the crown and roots

255. Avulsed teeth may be repositioned and stabilized in the dental arch by application of

(a) a splint
(b) stainless steel crowns
(c) polycarboxylate crowns
(d) a bite plane

256. Which of the following prostheses provides protection for the teeth during contact sports?

(a) removable partial denture
(b) bite plane
(c) mouth guard
(d) custom splint

257. When placing a stainless steel crown, how should a snug fit at the gingival margin of the preparation be obtained?

(a) reduce the circumference of the crown with crown shears at the facial-lingual area
(b) crimp the circumference inward with ball-and-socket–type pliers
(c) reduce the circumference of the crown at the mesial-distal area
(d) crimp the circumference outward at the mesial-distal only

258. A stainless steel crown is contoured at the

    (a) mesial only

    (b) distal only

    (c) gingival margin

    (d) mesial-distal contact areas

259. In pediatric dentistry, when is the use of varnish contraindicated?

    (a) before seating an amalgam

    (b) before use of zinc phosphate cement

    (c) before seating a stainless steel crown

    (d) under composite resins

260. The three types of matrix bands available for use in pediatric dentistry are

    (1) Tofflemire

    (2) T-band

    (3) spot-welded matrix

    (4) sprue band

    (5) plastic band

        (a) 1, 2, 3

        (b) 1, 3, 4

        (c) 2, 3, 4

        (d) 2, 4, 5

261. Which of the following materials is used to fill primary root canals?

    (a) calcium hydroxide

    (b) zinc phosphate

    (c) zinc oxide–eugenol

    (d) gutta percha

262. Which of the following figures provides for operating on the first molar?

    (a) A

    (b) B

    (c) A and B

    (d) neither A nor B

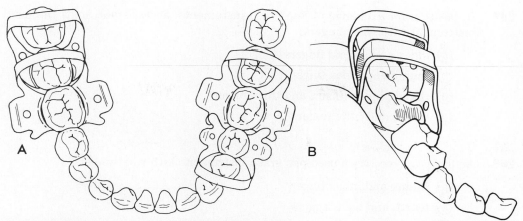

Piggyback clamps on first and second molars. (From Baum L, Phillips RW, Lund MR: The Textbook of Operative Dentistry, 2nd ed. Philadelphia, WB Saunders, 1985, p 192)

Molar clamps, second premolar clamp.

263. Which one of the following instruments used in the slow speed handpiece functions to spin filling materials into the canals?

    (a) Gates-Glidden bur

    (b) Peeso reamer

    (c) reamer with lateral attachment

    (d) lentulo spiral

264. Endodontic broaches are primarily used for

    (a) gross removal of soft tissue from the canal spaces of vital teeth

    (b) shaping root canals

    (c) enlarging root canals

    (d) planing intracanal walls

265. An endodontic explorer may be used for

    (a) holding gutta percha cones during heat transmission

    (b) condensing gutta percha

    (c) checking intracanal walls

    (d) locating canal orifices

266. Endodontic finger spreaders and pluggers differ in that pluggers

    (a) are flat at the ends

    (b) are used to obturate the canal

    (c) may be handled or finger type

    (d) are stainless steel that has not been annealed

267. In position for exchange of pen grasp instuments, an assistant holds the new instrument with what fingers?

    (a) index and second fingers

    (b) thumb and index finger

    (c) thumb, index finger, and third finger

    (d) fourth and little fingers

268. An assistant receives a used pen grasp instrument with what fingers?

    (a) thumb and index finger

    (b) fourth and little fingers

    (c) thumb, index and third fingers

    (d) index and second fingers

269. When flossing, care should be taken to avoid

    (a) removing a filling

    (b) injury to gingival tissues

    (c) using waxed floss

    (d) placing the floss through the contact areas

270. Amalgam may be used as a

    (1) Class II restoration

    (2) Class IV restoration

    (3) Class III restoration

    (4) core under a full crown

        (a) 1, 2

        (b) 1, 3

        (c) 1, 4

        (d) 2, 4

271. When loading an amalgam capsule, the correct ratio of alloy pellets to spills of mercury is

    (a) one pellet to one spill

    (b) two pellets to one spill

    (c) three pellets to two spills

    (d) two pellets to three spills

272. A Jo Dandy disk is included in the setup for what procedure?
    (a) coronal polish
    (b) polishing an inlay
    (c) cutting a metallic restoration
    (d) finishing a cavity preparation

273. A cuttlefish bone disk is included in the setup for finishing which of the following materials?
    (a) composite
    (b) glass ionomer
    (c) polycarboxylate
    (d) gold

274. Placing a matrix band too snugly around a tooth with a Class II preparation for an amalgam restoration could result in
    (a) overhanging margins
    (b) voids in the amalgam restoration
    (c) deficient contact areas
    (d) amalgam shrinkage

275. The term *attenuated* referring to microbial activity means
    (a) killed
    (b) diluted
    (c) weakened
    (d) strengthened

276. When requested to perform illegal procedures, a dental assistant should
    (a) indicate incapability to perform the procedure
    (b) submit resignation from employment
    (c) proceed to perform the function
    (d) explain the state law regulating performance by a dental assistant and refuse to perform the procedure

277. Expanded intraoral functions may legally be performed by an educated licensed auxiliary when
    (a) delegated to a dental auxiliary and supervised by a dentist
    (b) requested to prepare the teeth and place permanent restorations

Continued on next page

ⓒ the procedure is delegated by a dentist

ⓓ allowable according to state regulations and under a dentist's supervision

278. When a patient loses a gold crown and arrives at the dental office before the dentist returns from lunch, the chairside auxiliary

   ① advises the patient to wait
   ② checks the tooth for the extent of trauma
   ③ places a temporary crown
   ④ refers the patient to an oral surgeon
   ⑤ makes an appointment for the patient for the following week

   ⓐ 1 only
   ⓑ 4 only
   ⓒ 2, 3
   ⓓ 3, 5

279. While being seated and draped, a patient complains of pain and asks the chairside assistant to check the maxillary central incisor. The assistant does which of the following?

   ① notices whether the tooth is fractured
   ② states that the tooth should be extracted
   ③ makes a notation of the patient's complaint on the dental chart
   ④ states that the tooth should be prepared with a full porcelain-fused-to-metal crown
   ⑤ relates the information to the dentist

   ⓐ 1 only
   ⓑ 1, 3
   ⓒ 3, 5
   ⓓ 2, 4

280. Information that should be immediately gathered when a patient in pain telephones for an appointment includes

   ① how long the pain has continued
   ② whether the pain is constant or intermittent
   ③ if the patient has suffered nausea or vomiting
   ④ if the patient has any known allergies
   ⑤ if the patient has dental insurance

   ⓐ 1, 2
   ⓑ 1, 2, 3

(c) 1, 2, 3, 4

(d) 1, 2, 4, 5

281. When syncope occurs in a seemingly healthy patient, it should be assumed until proved otherwise that the unconsciousness represents

(a) hypertension

(b) hyperglycemia

(c) cardiac arrest

(d) local anesthetic agent toxic overdose

282. For a Class II three-surface restoration, the matrix band should extend occlusally

(a) 2 mm above the floor of the cavity preparation

(b) 1 to 2 mm above the marginal ridges of the tooth's complement in the same arch

(c) 1 to 2 mm above the marginal ridges of the opposing tooth

(d) 1 to 2 mm above the lingual and facial ridges

Rationale for
Test Questions

TEST I

Rationale for Test Questions
TEST I

ANSWERS AND RATIONALE

1. ⓒ To plan a safe and practical treatment schedule for a patient, it is essential to know the patient's most recent exposure to radiation, allergies and sensitivities, and routine medication.

2. ⓓ Basic vital signs considered essential for evaluating a patient's current state of health include respiration rate, pulse, temperature, and blood pressure.

3. ⓓ The pulse rate is measured in the radial artery of the wrist, where it is felt as a rhythmic expansion. The number of heart beats per minute represents the number of times that the heart contracts.

4. ⓑ The brachial artery is found in the antecubital fossa (indentation), in the curvature just above the inner portion of the lower arm.

5. ⓐ The average blood pressure of a healthy adult is approximately 120 *systolic* (pressure in the brachial artery) as the heart pumps the blood into the artery, over *70 diastolic* as the heart relaxes and takes blood into the right auricle, the upper right chamber of the heart.

6. ⓓ A woman's normal respiration rate when relaxing is 18 inhalations per minute; a man's normal respiration rate may be 16 to 17 inhalations per minute.

7. ⓒ The sequence of disinfecting the thermometer, storing it in a sterile container, and placing a disposable sleeve over it before inserting it in a patient's mouth is a procedure to protect patients from exposure to contamination.

8. ⓓ To read a thermometer quickly and effectively immediately after removing it from a patient's oral cavity, hold it at eye level and parallel to the floor, turn it slightly to see the extension of mercury, and read and record the number before the thermometer registers a temperature change.

9. ⓒ A clinical examination of the hard and soft tissues of the intraoral cavity includes the buccal mucosa, tongue, and palate. The commissures of the lips would be included in an extraoral examination.

10. ⓐ A clinical examination of the extraoral soft tissues includes kneading the lips between the fingers and thumb and visual examination of the philtrum and the vermilion border. Inspection of the labial frenum would be included in an *intraoral* examination.

11. (d) Tori of the palate and mandible are excess growths of bones. These growths are benign and may be removed surgically when they interfere with function or the fit of a prosthesis.

12. (c) A closed epithelium-lined sac containing liquid is a cyst walled off from the rest of the tissues. A pustule is an elevation of mucosa containing pus. An abscess is a localized collection of pus in a limited area (a sac). A vesicle could be described as blister-like in formation.

13. (d) An update on medications dispensed and ingested by a patient may have an effect on treatment considered by a dentist.

14. (d) Records are kept of analgesics because they may contain narcotics.

15. (d) When synergistic drugs are taken together, their individual effects are actually enhanced. Taken singly, the same drugs would not be so effective.

16. (c) Angina pectoris is a condition causing a contraction of the pericardium surrounding the heart. Chest pains are the result. Patients may be carrying nitroglycerin tablets to place under the tongue to relieve the distress by relaxing the heart muscle. Note: The mucosa under the tongue is conducive to the absorption of solid medication into the bloodstream.

17. (d) Iodophor solution and 2 percent glutaraldehyde solution are effective in sanitizing impressions as recommended by the Occupational Safety and Health Administration (OSHA) before forwarding them to the dental laboratory.

18. (b) Placing polysulfide elastomeric catalyst paste on the spatula before mixing aids in cleaning the spatula after the mix is loaded into the impression tray.

19. (d) Placing two coats of copal varnish on the dentin of a prepared tooth helps to avoid surface air bubbles and seals dentinal tubules.

20. (c) Temperature below the dew point of a glass slab deters the incorporation of moisture into the mix of dental cement.

21. (c) Using a warm, dry glass slab and rapidly spatulating the mix reduce the amount of cement powder that can be incorporated into the mix and shorten the setting time.

22. (d) Fluorides are present in glass ionomer cements.

23. (b) Isopropyl alcohol 70 percent placed on the tip of an instrument prevents cement from sticking to the instrument.

24. (a) Ethoxybenzoic acid (EBA) cement is mixed with a small spatula on a paper pad, similar to zinc oxide–eugenol cement.

25. (c) An automixer dispenser has two chambers for polysilicone-type impression material; squeezing the gun moves the plunger forward, forcing the pastes out the tip in a homogeneous mix.

26. (d) Overdrying the dentin (desiccation) causes sensitivity of the dentin. An imbalance of water content in the dentin may contribute to sensitivity and pulp pathology.

27. (b) Two drops of liquid to one scoop of powder provides the proper ratio for a mix of glass ionomer cement.

28. (d) A maximum mixing time of 40 seconds is adequate to achieve a satisfactory mix of glass ionomer cement for luting.

29. (a) One scoop of powder to one drop of liquid is adequate to achieve a thicker mix of glass ionomer cement for Class III and Class V restorations. Note: The mix needs to be thicker for a restoration than for luting.

30. (c) The dental cement compatible with all restorative dental materials is calcium hydroxide.

31. (a) Calcium hydroxide is the cement of choice to be placed in a tooth preparation with 1 mm or less of tooth structure over the pulp.

32. (c) Calcium hydroxide for liners in tooth preparations is available in two-paste, premixed, and light-cured systems.

33. (b) Varnishes may be placed in cavity preparations under composite restorations.

34. (d) To ensure etching and bonding of composites with the enamel, the polishing paste used to clean the tooth enamel must be free of fluorides.

35. (b) Zinc phosphate cement is frequently used to insulate a tooth in a deep preparation and for luting cast restorations.

36. (c) Zinc phosphate cement is not placed over the pulp of a deep preparation because acid in the liquid is irritating to the pulp.

37. (c) Vinyl polysiloxane, polyether, and reversible hydrocolloid impression materials all are capable of obtaining sharp detail of the margins of a tooth preparation for a cast restoration.

38. (d) A dentist is legally responsible for keeping an ongoing record of all drugs administered or prescribed for a patient.

39. (d) Parenteral drug administration literally means "by injection under the skin."

40. (b) Antihistamines are used to counteract the effect of any drugs that cause mild or severe allergic reactions in a patient.

41. (c) The *body* of a prescription begins with the R_x symbol and contains the name and strength of the drug prescribed. The *heading* includes information about the prescriber and the patient. The *closing* contains final instructions to the pharmacist, as well as the prescriber's signature.

42. (d) *Post cibum* (p.c) means "after meals," q.i.d. stands for "four times daily," b.i.d. indicates "twice daily," and p.r.n. stands for "as needed."

43. (a) Bacteria progress from a carious lesion to the pulp by way of the dentinal tubules.

44. (a) A barbed broach is an instrument used to initially enlarge the root canal in endodontic treatment. Broaches are primarily used for gross removal of soft tissue from the canal space of vital teeth and for removal of diseased pulp. Reamers with files are used for canal enlargement.

45. (d) Reamer sizes range from 10 to 140.

46. (c) The Glick #1 instrument was designed for placement of temporary fillings with the paddle end and removal of excess gutta percha with the plugger end.

47. (a) Debridement is the process of removing existing and potential irritants from the root canal.

48. (c) Sodium hypochlorite placed in a syringe is used to irrigate and cleanse the root canal. It is a solvent for necrotic tissue and is an effective disinfectant and bleach.

49. (b) Gutta percha is the most common neutral material used for obturation (closing) of a sterile root canal. Some disadvantages of silver points are that they cannot be adapted to irregularly shaped canals, they may be toxic, and their removal is difficult.

50. (a) Most sealer materials used in endodontics are zinc oxide–eugenol based. Plastics have desirable properties but are less available and more expensive than the zinc oxide-eugenol–based materials.

51. (c) Root canal sealers are mixed to a thick consistency to withstand condensing and packing of the canal and to fortify the tooth. The thicker the mix, the better the seal and the less toxicity.

52. (d) Gutta percha points are disinfected by placing individual points in cold chemical solutions such as glutaraldehydes before placement. Heat disinfection would melt the material.

53. (c) A parallel right-angle technique provides the most accurate radiographic projection of the long axis of a tooth.

54. (b) Hydrogen peroxide (3 percent) will effectively "bubble out" debris as it liberates free oxygen when contacting organic tissue. It does not need a lengthy time to react. It will partially disinfect the canal. However, preparations containing hydrogen peroxide should *never* be left in a canal because of their tendency to cause irritation by percolating out of the apex of the tooth into the surrounding tissues.

55. (c) Pulpectomy is surgical removal of a vital pulp within a tooth. The suffix *-ectomy* means "to remove." Pulpotomy is partial excision of the dental pulp.

56. (c) Chelators are placed after instruments have been used to mechanically remove infectious and organic debris from a canal.

57. (d) A root canal gun (Messing gun) is used to retrofill a prepared tooth after an apicoectomy. The material of choice is zinc-free silver alloy.

58. (b) Percussion of a tooth with inflamed or sensitive pulpal tissue is an effective diagnostic method. This gentle tapping may cause discomfort to patients.

59. (a) Hepatitis B virus concentrates in the dark, moist area of the gingival sulcus. Because in most patients' mouths this area is inflamed and easily allows blood to mix with saliva and crevicular fluid, operators who work in the area are at risk.

60. (c) Thorough cleansing of the surface of an object reduces the debris and microbial mass that contaminate. After cleansing, application of a disinfectant agent is advised. In the presence of accumulated bioburden, many chemical disinfectants lack effective antimicrobial activity.

61. (b) To sterilize instruments effectively, preliminary preparation must include removing gross debris and lubricating moving parts before autoclaving. During these procedures, an operator must wear protective barriers. Note: The detergent used should have a low pH.

62. (c) Bioburden is the mass of debris that is found on an instrument after its use. This debris must be removed because it inhibits the effectiveness of the sterilization process.

63. (d) Iodophors, sodium hypochlorite, and complex phenol agents are approved by the Centers for Disease Control for sanitation purposes.

64. (c) Clean-up procedures following dental treatment provide rapid action on the microbial mass and eliminate potential sources of cross-infection. Germicides used must penetrate into the crevices of equipment.

65. (a) A patient updated medical history provides a basis for a dentists' diagnosis and plan of treatment. All patients must be treated as though they are infectious disease risks.

66. (d) Because clinic attire becomes contaminated during the day, it should not be worn out of the workplace but should be removed for laundering. Clothing different from street clothes must be worn during treatment and must not be worn outside the workplace.

67. (a) A rubber dam is an excellent inhibitor to the spread of infectious materials.

68. (d) Exposure to infection by health care workers is usually due to being injured by contaminated syringe needles or surgical instruments (sharps). Sharps

include new or used hollow-nose needles, scalpels, blades, suture needles, pointed instruments, burs, glass, anesthetic Carpules, orthodontic wires, and others.

69. ⓓ Steam autoclaving is the recommended method of sterilization for contaminated handpieces. With this method, both the interior and exterior portions are sterilized.

70. ⓑ Bacterial spores are placed in monitors for determining the effectiveness of the sterilization process. These are more resistant to heat than are viruses and vegetative bacteria.

71. ⓐ For the sterilization process to be effective, instruments must be dry before being placed in a dry heat sterilizer.

72. ⓑ To prevent corrosion and rust, carbon steel instruments are treated with a corrosion inhibitor before steam autoclaving.

73. ⓐ Universal precautions dictate that all apparel worn by the dental team and contacted by body fluids must be discarded or laundered after a single use.

74. ⓑ To protect dental personnel and patients, overgloves are used when performing all secondary procedures. Overglove use is indicated when the provider will return to the same patient after treatment has been temporarily interrupted.

75. ⓒ Utility gloves may be scrubbed, decontaminated, and reused. Utility gloves are *not* used when providing treatment to patients.

76. ⓑ The office staff must use a surgical scrub to decontaminate gloved hands when returning to chairside.

77. ⓓ A wet mask is not effective and should be discarded; a protective mask barrier must be clean and dry.

78. ⓒ Boiling water is no longer an acceptable form of sterilization.

79. ⓑ To allow sufficient circulation of steam and heat under pressure, a large instrument pack should be placed on the bottom of the chamber of the steam autoclave. Otherwise, it would block the flow of steam.

80. ⓓ Sodium hypochlorite solution deteriorates quickly and must be freshly mixed on a daily basis.

81. ⓐ Glutaraldehydes produce toxic fumes.

82. ⓒ Ultrasonic cleaning solution should be changed daily. The solution should be discarded at the end of the day, and the inside of the pan and lids wiped with a cleaning and disinfecting solution.

83. ⓓ A muslin wrap of instruments for autoclaving permits the steam heat to penetrate into the material and sterilize the instruments. The material
Continued on next page

should be porous but should not have the type of holes created by pins or staples.

84. ⓓ For operator and patient protection, latex gloves should be worn when placing and exposing dental film for radiographs. In addition, the tube head should be protected with clear plastic barriers.

85. ⓒ Alginate impressions should be sprayed with a disinfecting agent immediately on removal from a patient's mouth. Immersion could cause distortion of the impression and is *not* advised.

86. ⓓ To prevent water and a patient's saliva from being sucked back into the dental unit, antiretraction valves must be installed. Without this device there is a potential for drawing water or saliva from one patient's procedure and then passing it into the mouth of the next patient.

87. ⓒ Regular antimicrobial hand washings aid in combating the increase of skin microbial growth. Residual activity becomes evident after the eighth hand wash of the day and builds throughout the continuing hand washes.

88. ⓑ For removal of spatter and contaminants, protective eye wear should be routinely cleaned between patients. Disinfection or sterilization of eye wear is difficult.

89. ⓓ Viruses causing influenza, the common cold, and hepatitis B can be transmitted through the conjunctiva of the eye.

90. ⓒ Most topical anesthetic ointments achieve effectiveness on tissues in 2 to 3 minutes.

91. ⓒ With the bevel of the needle turned toward the alveolus, the anesthetic solution is more readily deposited near the roots and nerves of the tooth.

92. ⓑ Epinephrine is a stimulant to the heart and is *not* recommended for a patient with a heart condition.

93. ⓒ For safety reasons, a needle guard is removed after a syringe is positioned in the operator's hand.

94. ⓑ When local anesthetic solutions turn amber color in the Carpule, they are too old and must be discarded.

95. ⓒ An assistant places an anesthetic syringe into an operator's hand, and the ring is fitted onto the operator's thumb.

96. ⓒ When an accidental needle stick occurs, make the injured tissue bleed to remove initial contaminants, rinse under running water, and swab the site with a disinfecting solution.

97. ⓑ A long syringe needle is indicated for local anesthetic solution injection of the inferior alveolar nerve.

98. (b) Because a patient loses consciousness during general anesthesia, throat packs and maintenance of the airway are mandatory.

99. (b) Patients must not eat 6 to 8 hours before general anesthesia is administered because food could be regurgitated, causing them to aspirate the food and choke.

100. (e) Herpes simplex virus (fever blisters and cold sores) may be dormant for years, lesions usually develop at the same site, and this virus may be transmitted through saliva.

101. (a) B complex vitamin deficiencies cause many systemic conditions, particularly pellagra, cheilosis, and glossitis. There is such a close interrelationship among the B complex vitamins that a deficiency of one impairs the utilization of the others.

102. (b) A biopsy is necessary to establish a definitive diagnosis for leukoplakia, which often precedes the development of a malignant tumor.

103. (d) The lymphatic system contains the cells responsible for immune responses of the body.

104. (d) Acetone breath, a rapid and weak pulse, and dry mouth are symptoms of hyperglycemia. Clammy skin, vertigo, sweating, and confusion are symptoms of hypoglycemia.

105. (c) The most resistant forms of bacteria are the type that go into a spore stage.

106. (b) Viruses are capable of multiplying only in living cell tissues.

107. (d) The ability to develop antibodies in the blood provides an individual with immunity. Antibodies are substances developed by the body in response to the presence of antigens.

108. (d) Thrombin and tannic acid promote the clotting of blood.

109. (b) If coronary arteries become blocked, the result is myocardial infarction. The coronary arteries supply blood to the heart muscle, and a blockage can result in the death of a portion of the heart muscle.

110. (a) If a victim has an insufficient amount of oxygen in the blood reaching the brain, the pupils are dilated when exposed to light. If the tissues are not receiving oxygen, blood is not circulating.

111. (a) Dextrose 50 percent should be provided intravenously for a patient suffering from a hypoglycemic coma, which indicates a low glucose content of the blood. The patient should also be positioned for shock and for possible oxygen administration.

112. (b) The head tilt is necessary to maintain a free airway during use of an Ambu bag.

113. (d) A choking patient is directed to keep the mouth open during administration of the Heimlich maneuver.

114. (a) The abdominal thrust may be used to dislodge an object in the airway of a conscious patient.

115. (c) First aid for a patient suffering a heart attack includes calling 911 for paramedics, keeping the victim quiet and comfortable, and administering 100 percent oxygen.

116. (d) All of the measures listed in the question are appropriate if a patient is in pulmonary arrest and has ceased breathing.

117. (e) Abdominal thrust, mouth-to-mouth, and mouth-to-nose artificial ventilation are acceptable, depending on the extent and location of an injury.

118. (b) A patient is given one breath to five chest compressions when a two-rescuer CPR team is working.

119. (b) Reduce the pressure for chest compression and the force of artificial ventilation when performing CPR on an infant or small child.

120. (c) Reversible hydrocolloid needs to be conditioned in an airtight container placed in a boiling water bath.

121. (c) Monies owed by the dental practice are *accounts payable* (the cost of the practice).

122. (e) Fixed overhead includes those expenses that are constant month after month.

123. (b) One method to create space for impression material when fabricating a custom tray is to use two layers of base plate wax over the cast.

124. (a) PSL-polysiloxane impression material comes in light, regular, and heavy-bodied consistency.

125. (e) The elastomeric group of impression materials are composed of a base and a catalyst.

126. (a) Reversible hydrocolloid impressions provide sharp detail of the prepared teeth. They are likely to tear when removed from deep undercuts and should be handled with care.

127. (c) Holes cut into the base plate wax covering a stone cast provide for "stops" within a custom tray.

128. (a) A back order is notice from a supply house that a particular item is out of stock and will be delivered later.

129. (b) Supplies that are used and replaced are referred to as *expendable items*.

130. ⓒ The name of the person who writes the check (payor) is not included in the check register.

131. ⓐ When checks are canceled by the bank, the amount is deducted from the checking account.

132. ⓐ A check for $16.83 will replenish the petty cash fund.

133. ⓐ

134. ⓒ Quarterly reports are required of taxable wages paid to each employee.

135. ⓑ Adding additional monies to the original amount of a check by anyone other than the payor is referred to as *raising a check*.

136. ⓔ Triturating correctly and placing, condensing, and carving a silver amalgam restoration while the material is pliable are essential. The assistant and operator must also be careful to avoid contamination of the mass of silver amalgam.

137. ⓒ A T band, Tofflemire band, and wedged metal strip all serve as acceptable matrices when placing a Class II amalgam restoration. A T band is a custom matrix band that is adaptable to a prepared primary tooth. Spot-welded matrices may also be used.

138. ⓒ An acceptable matrix for an amalgam restoration must be flexible and easy to apply.

139. ⓒ A posterior three-quarter crown would *not* cover the facial surface (for aesthetic purposes).

140. ⓓ Pontics and abutments are units of a fixed bridge. Clasps and rests are also considered to be units.

141. ⓑ A retention pin to be located for each cusp of the crown is usually indicated.

142. ⓑ The strength of a maxillary cuspid is ensured with three pins, mesial distal area of the facial surface, and the cingulum.

143. ⓓ Amalgam, reinforced glass ionomer, and composites are used for crown core build-ups.

144. ⓑ Racemic epinephrine is a vascular constrictor and a stimulant to the heart; therefore, it is not used in retraction cord for patients with cardiovascular disease.

145. ⓑ Adequate time for retraction of the gingiva on a preparation is 5 to 7 minutes. Time is dependent on the type of chemical retraction used.

146. ⓒ Retraction cord is packed in a clockwise direction and removed in a counterclockwise direction. The cord is overlapped where the ends meet.

147. ⓒ Stops in custom trays provide adequate space for impression material. When taking an impression, the tray stops at a particular position, preventing setting the tray too deep onto the dental arch.

148. ⓑ Temporary aluminum crowns should extend approximately 0.5 mm beyond the gingival margin of the prepared tooth.

149. ⓓ The sprue in a wax pattern should be placed at the heaviest area of the pattern, away from the margins, to avoid weakening of the pattern and distortion of the margins.

150. ⓐ The genial tubercles are lingual to the mandibular centrals.

151. ⓑ Post damming in a maxillary denture is located in the areas of a patient's transverse palatine suture.

152. ⓓ After the extraction of teeth, the alveolar ridge resorbs, thus creating a need to reline an immediate denture in order to reobtain a snug fit.

153. ⓒ Dental plaque is composed of food debris, epithelial cells, and mucin. If left untouched, the accumulation contributes to the development of caries and periodontal disease.

154. ⓒ Patients should learn the steps of plaque prevention and control procedures. A part of this is conscientious home care, which certainly can help to diminish the development of plaque, stain, and calculus.

155. ⓐ It is understood that chronic gingivitis is caused by local irritants such as accumulated plaque, calcareous deposits (tartar), and so on.

156. ⓒ A periodontal pack placed after surgery protects the wound, alleviates discomfort, aids healing, and supports teeth that are mobile until bony support occurs.

157. ⓒ After surgery, patients are advised to increase their intake of fluids, avoid chewing on hard foods, and contact the office if swelling is long lasting or painful. A small amount of bleeding is not a reason for concern.

158. ⓑ After removal of a periodontal surgical pack, patients are advised to use dental floss or tape cautiously and to irrigate the interproximal areas using warm water.

159. ⓐ To control the right-angle handpiece during a coronal polishing procedure, a fulcrum and pen grasp are used.

160. ⓓ A polishing strip is used interproximally to remove stains from anterior teeth.

161. ⓒ During a coronal polishing procedure, bristle brushes are used in the handpiece to remove stains from the occlusal surfaces of the teeth.

162. ⓐ Burnishers are not applicable to periodontal treatment or surgery.

163. (d) The coronal polishing procedure setup calls for a slow-speed handpiece; a high-speed handpiece would create friction and heat.

164. (a) Abrading enamel at the cervical area of a tooth develops into a wedge-shaped depression.

165. (c) A dentist may apply tinted sealants to detect more readily the retention of the material on the occlusal anatomy of the tooth.

166. (c) During surgical procedures, a rongeur is used to remove sharp edges and to promote a smoother surface of the alveolar crest.

167. (a) After oral surgery, cold, dry packs are applied intermittently to the facial surface for the first 24 hours to control swelling.

168. (d) If a blood clot is dislodged from the socket after an extraction, the opening in the alveolus is exposed, causing pain for the patient.

169. (d) The organic type of suture that is absorbed by the body during the healing process is gut suture.

170. (a) Hand scrubbing is the first step in the aseptic technique for the dental team before performing oral surgery.

171. (a) The exolever surgical instrument is designed to elevate an impacted tooth from its socket.

172. (c) Peanuts, pretzels, and popcorn are the foods least likely to be cariogenic as snack food.

173. (c) Sugar-free gelatins and soft drinks are low in caloric content and nutrients.

174. (a) Complex carbohydrates, such as complex starches, serve as the major source of energy for most people.

175. (b) Proteins are essential nutrients that provide the fundamental structural element of every cell.

176. (d) Oxygen is the most effective agent for resuscitative procedures as dictated by the emergency.

177. (c) Nitrous oxide and oxygen produce relative analgesia and reduce apprehension and fear for patients.

178. (e) Nitrous oxide and oxygen are not indicated as relative analgesia for patients with respiratory problems or if it is difficult to communicate with the patient. These patients may not be able to cooperate or to understand a procedure.

179. (b) An assistant always functions under the direct supervision of a dentist when assisting in administering nitrous oxide and oxygen, including monitoring the tanks.

180. ⓓ When baseline values are achieved, the patient and nitrous oxide–oxygen equipment are monitored continuously by the dental team.

181. ⓒ When a patient becomes alert after administration of nitrous oxide–oxygen, the mask is removed, the chair back is slowly lifted, and the baseline for the patient is recorded on the chart.

182. ⓒ The prevent a needle stick, an assistant must place the used needle into the open end of a cover guard *before* it is removed from the used syringe.

183. ⓒ Reversible-type impression materials such as reversible hydrocolloid may be used for construction of complete dentures and implants.

184. ⓓ Irreversible hydrocolloid impression materials such as alginates may be used for constructing opposing arch and study casts.

185. ⓒ Impression materials used to obtain bite registrations include zinc oxide–eugenol impression pastes and elastomers such as the vinyl polysiloxanes.

186. ⓒ Type II gypsum material used for dental casts is referred to as *model plaster.*

187. ⓑ Type IV gypsum is referred to as *high-strength, improved, densite dental stone.* It is denser in structure than model or impression plaster.

188. ⓐ The Type IV stone formula is 22 ml of water to 100 grams of powder.

189. ⓒ Silver amalgam filling material is composed of silver filings, titanium, and copper mixed with mercury.

190. ⓒ Disadvantages of silver amalgam include its high rate of thermal conductivity, its failure to bond with tooth dentin and enamel, its tendency to tarnish when not polished, and the need for bulk to provide strength.

191. ⓑ To reduce exposure of dental personnel to mercury vapors, silver amalgam is precapsulated, mixed in a covered amalgamator, and dispensed into the cavity preparation without touching human tissues.

192. ⓐ The synthetic resins frequently used for construction of custom temporary coverage self-polymerize.

193. ⓐ To ligate a rubber dam, a length of dental floss may be doubled and placed interproximally at the tooth opposite the anchor tooth. This serves to stabilize the dam.

194. ⓑ A Young frame may be used to mechanically hold a rubber dam away from the face.

195. ⓐ When placing a rubber dam over a three-unit fixed bridge, the punch hole for the anchor tooth is larger and the facial and lingual punch holes are made near the unclamped abutment to the fixed bridge. No hole is punched for the pontic, and the facial and lingual holes are positioned near the mesial surface of the pontic to aid in ligation of an anchor tooth.

196. ⓒ Attempts are made to reconstruct the configuration of a rubber dam after its removal from the oral cavity. The operator checks carefully for torn fragments, tears, and the cut septa to be certain that all dam tissue is accounted for.

197. ⓒ Zinc phosphate cement may be used as an insulating base within a preparation and for luting (cementing) a cast restoration.

198. ⓒ Because zinc phosphate cement is irritating to the pulpal tissues of the teeth, it is not placed near the pulp in a deep preparation; however, it does provide good adherence when margins are not exposed.

199. ⓐ Zinc phosphate cement is commonly placed over calcium hydroxide to serve as an insulating base.

200. ⓑ Instrumentation for zinc phosphate includes a cool, dry glass slab and dispensers for the powder and liquid as well as a flexible steel spatula.

201. ⓓ Acceptable zinc phosphate cement mixes for cementation must hang in a syrupy drop 1 inch from the spatula.

202. ⓑ An acceptable method of slightly retarding the setting of zinc phosphate cement mix is to incorporate a very small amount of powder into the liquid, let it set for 15 seconds, then continue the mixing process until a medium syrupy mix is obtained.

203. ⓑ Zinc oxide – eugenol is effective when used for a temporary restoration, as a palliative for tooth tissues, and as an insulating base placed over calcium hydroxide.

204. ⓒ A mix of zinc oxide – eugenol cement for temporary coverage should be of medium thickness, and free flowing, and it should set in no more than 5 minutes.

205. ⓒ The chemical therapeutic method of choice to control caries is the use of fluorides. This is enhanced by regular brushing, coronal polishing, and the use of plaque retardants.

206. ⓓ To restore a Class IV fracture of an anterior tooth, the materials of choice would be calcium hydroxide for the pulpal area and microfilled composite as the restorative material.

207. ⓑ The length of the blade is the second number in a three-number formula.

208. ⓑ To ensure safety and control of a rubber dam clamp, an operator positions the lingual jaws first, followed by the facial jaws. This mode of placement also affords a view of the clamp jaws as they are set.

209. (d) The beaver-tail burnisher is a favored instrument for inversion of the margin of the rubber dam.

210. (c) Use of the anterior portion of the opposite arch as a fulcrum point during examination of a maxillary central is acceptable.

211. (d) Using the ring finger as a fulcrum, the thumb, forefinger, and the end of the middle finger stabilize the handpiece when polishing the occlusal surface of the mandibular left first molar or other molars.

212. (c) Plastic type and amalgam fillings are polished using various sizes of grit on abrasive tools (e.g., sandpaper, carborundum, garnet, and cuttlefish bone).

213. (b) Hoes are beveled on the back of the cutting edge and must be used in a scraping action. Scraping may be toward the operator or from side to side.

214. (c) When working on the mandible, the fulcrum is established by the ring finger (fourth finger).

215. (b) Mild soap or shaving cream may be used as a lubricant on the tissue side of a rubber dam before placement. The lubricant should be water soluble because oil penetrates and can quickly rot the dam.

216. (c) It is advisable to expose at least seven teeth when applying an anterior rubber dam. This number of teeth provides for stability of the dam and adequate space for placement of at least one or two dam clamps. An operator has access, the lips are reflected, and the number of dry teeth is adequate to provide finger rests.

217. (b) The rubber dam napkin is placed next to the face under the rubber dam to provide comfort for a patient. The dam is left free to allow for napkin placement.

218. (d) A #212 Ferrier clamp is routinely used to isolate the cervical area of a tooth for a Class V preparation.

219. (a) The inner nut of a Tofflemire retainer is turned clockwise to make the retainer loop smaller. The inner nut controls the position of the vise to open and close the band.

220. (c) The assistant is positioned 4 to 6 inches above the level of the operator when working as a team in four-handed dentistry. With the patient reclining, the assistant's hips should be level with the patient's shoulders.

221. (a) The operator should be at the 12 o'clock position when working on the lingual surface of a patient's anterior maxillary teeth. The indirect technique is applied, viewing the tooth surfaces in a mouth mirror.

222. (d) When passing an anesthetic syringe to the operator, the assistant turns the bevel of the anesthetic syringe needle toward the alveolus (bone) in anticipation of correct placement for the operator's administration of local anesthetic solution.

223. (c) Below the patient's chin at the upper area of the chest is the instrument transfer zone.

224. (c) The Tanner and the Hollenback carvers and the burnishers are instruments used for providing detail on restorative material.

225. (b) The overhand grasp is the most versatile position when directing the high-velocity evacuation tip in four-handed dentistry. A reverse palm-thumb grasp is also often used.

226. (c) When final occlusal adjustments to amalgam and composite restorations are necessary, a rubber dam may be removed.

227. (c) The most commonly used rubber dam frames are the Young and the Woodbury.

228. (d) Silica-filled composite resins produce a smooth surface when cured, placed, and polished.

229. (a) Gel-type etchants are left in contact with the clean, dry enamel approximately 15 seconds.

230. (b) To determine that pit and fissure sealants are still intact on etched enamel, patients are recalled at 6-month intervals.

231. (c) Composite resins adapt to cast gold and bonded enamel veneer restorations.

232. (a) After rinsing and drying, properly etched tooth enamel should appear frosty white or satiny.

233. (d) Most enamel sealants are cured for 10 to 20 seconds per tooth using a curing light.

234. (b) Preparation of teeth for pit and fissure sealants may include the use of a soft prophy brush, fluoride-free abrasives, and possibly a #10 round bur to reduce the high areas after curing of the pit and fissure sealant.

235. (a) After the tooth surfaces have been cleaned, rinsed, and dried, the etching liquid or gel is applied and left for 15 to 30 seconds, depending on the manufacturer's recommendation.

236. (c) The maxillary molars are most frequently moved by extraoral headgear-type anchorage. This is done when the maxillary first molars are anteriorly positioned and the maxilla is growing rapidly.

237. (d) In intramaxillary anchorage, the resistance units involved in orthodontic treatment are confined to one arch. This involves the use of a removable appliance with secured springs and screws.

238. (d) Brackets are directly bonded to etched tooth enamel by applying composite resin to the base of the bracket.

239. (a) An adaptable instrument for removing bonded brackets from the teeth is the pin and ligature cutter, which is applied to the bracket at the margins and base and twisted.

240. (b) to efficiently remove a steel spring separator, an instrument is placed in the helix and the separator is carefully lifted upward away from the tooth. Caution is needed to avoid snapping the separator off of the tooth and causing it to fly out of control. A standard scaler may be used here.

241. (d) Posterior molars are selected for seating of bands with buccal tubes. The tubes receive extensions of the arch wire.

242. (d) The Boone gauge is the instrument used to determine the position of the bands on anterior teeth. The distance between the top edge of the band and the incisal edge is measured.

243. (d) Habitually thrusting the tongue against the anterior maxillary teeth may cause an open bite over a prolonged period of time. Thumb or finger sucking can also cause an open bite.

244. (d) A custom or stock space maintainer may be placed in the area of missing teeth to maintain the space for teeth erupting at a later date.

245. (d) The palm thumb grasp is recommended when using the ligature-tying pliers. They are held in the palm with the thumb placed between the handles and resting on the center post at the joint.

246. (c) Three different attachments may be soldered on a maxillary molar band as treatment modality dictates: an arch wire tube, a headgear tube, and a lingual cleat.

247. (b) Generally, removal of bands may require the use of band removal pliers, the Schure instrument, and a heavy-duty scaler. How pliers are used to adapt ligature wires.

248. (c) During a coronal polishing procedure, a soft-bristled brush and a mild abrasive are used with a right-angle handpiece to polish the occlusal surfaces.

249. (d) To stabilize the right-angle handpiece during a coronal polishing procedure, the fulcrum is established on the incisal edges of anteriors, occlusal surfaces of posteriors, or near the teeth in the same quadrant, depending on the teeth to be polished.

250. (d) In some instances, during a coronal polishing procedure, the hand directing the handpiece may establish stability on the chin of the patient or by forming a fulcrum near the area to be polished.

251. (c) A coronal polishing procedure is accomplished using a lifting, sweeping, and stroking motion when directing the right-angle handpiece.

252. ⓑ The goal of a coronal polishing procedure is to remove plaque and extrinsic stains.

253. ⓓ Abrasive materials for a coronal polishing procedure should mix readily to make a slurry with a fluoride base.

254. ⓓ A pulpectomy is a surgical procedure removing the pulpal tissues in the crown and roots of a tooth. A pulpotomy is removal of the coronal pulp.

255. ⓐ Teeth that are traumatized and displaced from the oral cavity may be repositioned and stabilized using a custom splint. The splint protects fractured, loosened, or avulsed teeth in the alveolus.

256. ⓒ Athletes competing in contact sports should wear custom mouth guards to protect their teeth.

257. ⓑ Crimping the circumference of a stainless steel crown inward with ball-and-socket pliers produces a snug fit on the crown.

258. ⓓ A stainless steel crown is contoured at the mesial-distal contact areas, thus making contact with adjacent teeth in the arch.

259. ⓓ Copal or synthetic varnish is contraindicated when using composite resins. It prevents the composite from reaching a final set.

260. ⓐ Tofflemire, T-band, and spot-welded custom bands are used in pediatric dentistry.

261. ⓒ Zinc oxide–eugenol is used to fill the canals of primary teeth.

262. ⓒ

263. ⓓ A lentulo spiral is a twisted wire instrument placed in a slow-speed handpiece. It spins filling material into prepared root canals.

264. ⓐ Endodontic broaches remove gross soft tissue and debris from canals of vital teeth.

265. ⓓ An endodontic explorer aids in locating orifices (openings) of root canals. It may also be used as a diagnostic aid to stimulate carious dentin as a test for responsiveness.

266. ⓐ Pluggers are flat at the ends to provide more force for condensing plastic filling material in sterile canals. Spreaders are pointed.

267. ⓒ In four-handed dentistry, an assistant holds the new instrument with the thumb, index finger, and third finger while extending the little finger to receive the used instrument from the operator. The shaft of the new instrument is grasped above its center.

268. ⓑ An assistant receives a pen grasp instrument with the fourth and little fingers.

269. (b) Avoid snapping floss through the contacts and injuring the gingival papilla. Care should be taken to ease the floss between the contacts of the teeth.

270. (c) Amalgam restorations may be used for Class II, Class I, or Class V and to build a core under a full crown preparation.

271. (a) If manually dispensing amalgam alloy and mercury, the recommended ratio is one pellet of alloy to one spill of mercury (1:1).

272. (c) A Jo Dandy, a carborundum disk, is used to cut metallic restorations or enamel tooth structure.

273. (d) Cuttlefish bone abrasive is included in the setup to polish a gold casting.

274. (c) Contouring of a matrix band must be sufficient to provide adequate contact with the adjacent teeth. A loose gingival margin would allow for overhangs or failure to protect the interproximal gingiva.

275. (c) In the study of infectious diseases, the term *attenuated* describes the state of microbes as being weakened. Weakening a virulent microbe or virus can prepare it for inclusion in the preparation of materials used for acquired immunization (e.g., the influenza virus attenuated in the flu vaccine).

276. (d) Dental assistants and other dental auxiliaries are limited to performing dental procedures described by the dental practice act of the state. The functions delegated are legal if indicated by the dental practice act or rules and regulations and if performed under the supervision of a dentist.

277. (d) A state's dental practice act must authorize and a dentist must delegate and supervise the performance of a specific dental procedure by a dental auxiliary when expanded intraoral functions are legal in that state.

278. (a) A dental auxiliary advises an emergency patient to await the dentist's return to the office. If the dentist is not in the dental office for the day, a patient should be immediately referred to the dental office where a reciprocal referral arrangement has been established. An auxiliary may in some states provide specific treatment procedures with the permission and under the supervision of a dentist.

279. (c) A dental auxiliary should at no time make a statement or give an opinion about a patient's condition, whether or not the patient has requested that the auxiliary inspect a tooth or the condition of the oral cavity. The auxiliary must listen attentively at all times for symptoms offered by the patient and record the comments for the dentist to evaluate or diagnose. An auxiliary must *not* offer diagnostic opinion; to do so is illegal and would constitute negligence and malpractice.

280. (a) Information helpful to a dentist would include the location of pain; how long it has continued; if there is a fever or swelling; if the pain is constant or intermittent; how the pain responds to hot, cold, sweets, and pressure; and whether or not there has been recent treatment or injury in the area.

281. ⓒ Syncope (fainting, unconsciousness) occurs in a seemingly healthy person when blood flow to the brain stops for an average of 6.8 seconds. It is the presenting sign of sudden death and implies cardiac arrest.

282. ⓑ The matrix bands should extend 1 to 2 mm above the marginal ridges, which can best be assessed by examining the complementary tooth in the same arch or an adjacent tooth in the arch. They should extend at least 1 mm beyond the gingival margin of the preparation to achieve an appropriate fit.

TEST II

General Dental Assisting — Advanced

TEST II

1. When compiling a patient's health history, it is appropriate to ask patients about
   1. regular medications taken
   2. congenital conditions
   3. chronic illnesses
   4. exposure to ionizing radiation
   5. adverse reactions to local or general anesthesia
      (a) 1 and 3
      (b) 2 and 4
      (c) 1, 2, 3
      (d) all of the above

2. Which of the following is essential when measuring a patient's blood pressure?
   (a) place the sphygmomanometer on the radial artery
   (b) place the disk of the stethoscope on the antecubital fossa
   (c) place the index and third finger on the brachial artery
   (d) inflate the cuff 50 points above average systolic pressure
   (e) deflate the cuff rapidly to obtain systole and diastole

3. Which of the following is essential to obtain an accurate temperature reading of a patient when using an oral mercury thermometer?
   (a) shake the mercury down into the bulb of the thermometer after removing the thermometer from the mouth

Continued on next page

(b) obtain the reading immediately after removing the thermometer from the oral cavity

(c) leave the thermometer under the tongue approximately 10 minutes

(d) rinse the patient's oral cavity with an antiseptic solution before inserting the thermometer

4. Which of the following are contagious lesions of the oral cavity?

(1) herpes simplex virus type 1 (HSV-1)

(2) aphthous ulcer (canker sore)

(3) herpes simplex virus type 2 (HSV-2)

(4) cheilosis

(5) linea alba

(a) 1, 3

(b) 2, 4

(c) 1, 2, 3

(d) all of the above

5. The teeth are attached to the bone in the absence of the periodontium in the condition known as

(a) cementosis

(b) anachoresis

(c) ankylosis

(d) arthropyosis

6. Which of the following can be very important in the development and progression of root caries?

(a) decreased salivary function

(b) surface hardness of enamel

(c) sulcus depth

(d) nursing bottles

7. How many schedules of pharmaceutical substances are controlled by the Federal Comprehensive Drug Abuse Prevention and Control Act of 1970?

(a) 3

(b) 4

(c) 5

(d) 6

8. Schedule II drugs that have accepted medical usefulness include

① opium

② morphine

③ codeine

④ barbiturates

⑤ aspirin

  ⓐ 1, 3

  ⓑ 2, 4

  ⓒ 1, 2, 3

  ⓓ 3, 4, 5

9. Which of the following is permissible by law when dispensing medications to patients in a dental office?

① controlled substances are personally dispensed by dentists

② patients are handed the substance, and staff may leave

③ dentists direct dental assistants to dispense specific medication under their supervision

④ dental assistants may be directed to administer a specific medication without the presence of a dentist

  ⓐ 1 only

  ⓑ 1, 3

  ⓒ 2, 4

  ⓓ 4 only

10. The objective in mixing the base and catalyst of silicone, polyether, and polysulfide impression materials is to obtain

  ⓐ a uniform cure of the mix

  ⓑ curing with less chair time

  ⓒ prolongation of curing time

  ⓓ absence of tissue irritation

11. Custom or stock trays may be used for elastomer-type impressions as long as

① peripheral wax is used

② tray adhesive is used

③ the tray is nonperforated

④ the tray is rimlocked

  ⓐ 1 only

  ⓑ 2 only

Continued on next page

ⓒ 1, 2

ⓓ 1, 3, 4

12. Which of the following applies to the placement of zinc oxide–eugenol cement when used for an insulating base?

    ⓐ it is mixed to a puttylike consistency

    ⓑ the mix covers the pulpal floor of the preparation

    ⓒ it is placed over a liner of calcium hydroxide

    ⓓ the mix is placed on the floor and dentinal walls of the cavity preparation

13. The material to aid in reducing microleakage between the margins of the enamel and a metallic restoration is

    ⓐ copal varnish

    ⓑ calcium hydroxide

    ⓒ glass ionomer cement

    ⓓ carboxylate cement

14. Which of the following dental materials insulate the pulp of a prepared tooth from thermal shock?

    ① zinc oxide–eugenol

    ② light-cured glass ionomers

    ③ carboxylates

    ④ synthetic resins

        ⓐ 1, 3

        ⓑ 2, 4

        ⓒ 1, 2, 3

        ⓓ 2, 3, 4

15. Which of the following materials is recognized as an insulator when placed directly over a traumatized pulp?

    ⓐ zinc phosphate cement

    ⓑ glass ionomer cement

    ⓒ calcium hydroxide

    ⓓ zinc oxide–eugenol

16. To restore a tooth with a vital traumatized pulp, the materials listed below would be used in what sequence?

① polycarboxylate cement
② cavity varnish
③ calcium hydroxide
④ silver amalgam
⑤ zinc oxide – eugenol

   ⓐ 2, 3, 1, 5, 4
   ⓑ 3, 2, 5, 1, 4
   ⓒ 5, 2, 3, 1, 4
   ⓓ 5, 3, 2, 1, 4

17. Which of the following cements are effective for luting orthodontic appliances to teeth?

① silicate
② silicophosphate
③ zinc oxide – eugenol
④ polycarboxylate

   ⓐ 1, 3
   ⓑ 2, 4
   ⓒ 1, 2, 3
   ⓓ 4 only

18. The glass ionomer generic formulas have been adapted for dentistry as

① luting agents
② cavity liners
③ Class I and Class II restorations
④ core build-up materials
⑤ light-cured systems

   ⓐ 1, 3
   ⓑ 2, 4
   ⓒ 3, 5
   ⓓ all of the above

19. Ethoxybenzoic acid (EBA) cement may be indicated for permanent cementation of inlays, crowns, and bridges because

① zinc oxide in the powder is nonirritating to sensitive teeth
② the mix reduces postoperative sensitivity of the tooth
③ the acid in the liquid increases the strength of the mix

Continued on next page

④ it reduces microleakage at the interface of the casting margins and the enamel

    ⓐ 1, 3

    ⓑ 2, 4

    ⓒ 1, 2, 3

    ⓓ 4 only

20. Which of the following is true of polycarboxylate (polyacrylate) cement?

    ① it is referred to as carboxylate cement

    ② the powder contains modified zinc oxide

    ③ the powder contains magnesium oxide

    ④ it may be placed under amalgam or composite restorations

       ⓐ 1, 3

       ⓑ 2, 3, 4

       ⓒ 4 only

       ⓓ all of the above

21. Visible light–activated elastomer impression material is a single component system available in formulas that

    ① are light bodied

    ② are heavy bodied

    ③ have catalytic function

       ⓐ 1 only

       ⓑ 1, 2

       ⓒ 1, 3

       ⓓ 2, 3

22. Glass ionomer cement is formulated for use in cementation of

    ① cast posts and cores

    ② orthodontic bands

    ③ cast crowns

    ④ custom temporary coverage

       ⓐ 1, 3

       ⓑ 2, 4

       ⓒ 1, 2, 3

       ⓓ 4 only

23. Which of the following is a function of glass ionomer cement?

    ⓐ periodontal splints

    ⓑ post and core build-up

    ⓒ Class IV anterior restoration

    ⓓ Class III anterior restoration

24. Which of the following steps are taken to prepare the capsule of glass ionomer cement?

    ① twist the knob end of the capsule

    ② place the capsule in the amalgamator for 10 seconds

    ③ place the capsule in a hand-held applicator

    ④ squeeze the mix into the tooth preparation

        ⓐ 1, 3

        ⓑ 2, 4

        ⓒ 1, 3, 4

        ⓓ 3, 4

25. When calcium hydroxide cement is used as an insulating base, the mix is placed

    ① level with the axial wall

    ② level with the pulpal wall

    ③ into the indentations of the preparation

    ④ to cover the margins of the preparation

        ⓐ 1, 2

        ⓑ 1, 3

        ⓒ 1, 2, 3

        ⓓ 2, 3, 4

26. In preparation for mixing zinc phosphate cement, the glass slab and spatula should be

    ⓐ dry and 68°F

    ⓑ dry and 72°F

    ⓒ moist and 74°F

    ⓓ moist and 76°F

27. Cavity varnishes composed of one or more resins in an organic solvent may be applied

    ① over a deep cavity preparation, before the insulating base

    ② over bases containing calcium hydroxide or zinc oxide–eugenol

Continued on next page

③ under a base of calcium hydroxide

④ to the base of the preparation only

    ⓐ 1 only

    ⓑ 2 only

    ⓒ 1, 2

    ⓓ 3, 4

28. Which of the following is applied to dentin to achieve maximum bonding when placing a glass ionomer restorative material?

    ⓐ 10 percent polyacrylic acid

    ⓑ light-cured zinc oxide–eugenol

    ⓒ 40 percent phosphoric acid

    ⓓ hydrogen peroxide

29. Which of the following may be used to retract the gingival tissue surrounding the finish line of a tooth prepared for a cast restoration?

① #212 cervical clamp

② rubber dam

③ stick compound

④ braided cord

    ⓐ 1, 3

    ⓑ 2, 4

    ⓒ 1, 2, 3

    ⓓ 4 only

30. A bite registration may be obtained using which of the following impression materials?

① vinyl polysiloxane

② alginic acid

③ wax with metallic filings

④ sticky peripheral wax

    ⓐ 1, 3

    ⓑ 2, 4

    ⓒ 3, 4

    ⓓ 4 only

31. One of the most common signs of the deterioration of a drug is a change in its

    ⓐ viscosity

(b) odor

(c) color

(d) molecular composition

32. Oral signs of drug abuse may include

(1) dry mouth

(2) rampant dental decay

(3) dental attrition

(4) periodontal disease

(a) 1, 2, 3

(b) 1, 2, 4

(c) 1, 3

(d) 2, 3, 4

(e) 1, 2, 3, 4

33. Which one of the following is an antifungal agent?

(a) nystatin

(b) cephalosporin

(c) erythromycin

(d) ampicillin

34. Which of the following statements correctly describe the procedure for ordering narcotics for the office supply?

(a) orders must be sent to the Drug Enforcement Administration

(b) a prescription must be completed for the local pharmacy so that it may fill the order

(c) a special opium supply order blank issued by the Bureau of Narcotics must be completed

(d) a copy of any order must be mailed to the Bureau of Narcotics

35. Which of the following condensers may be used to pack permanent root canal filling material?

(1) lateral

(2) vertical

(3) end

(4) Wesco

(a) 1, 3

(b) 2, 4

Continued on next page

ⓒ 4 only

ⓓ all of the above

36. What is the proper sequence for the use of a transistorized pulp vitalometer

① isolate the tooth to be tested with cotton rolls and dry

② begin the test with the rheostat set at zero

③ apply prophy paste to the facial or lingual surface of the tooth

④ place the conductive tip on the middle of the facial or lingual surface

⑤ increase the current rapidly if the conductive tip is placed on filling material

ⓐ 1, 3, 4, 2

ⓑ 1, 3, 2

ⓒ 2, 3, 4, 5

ⓓ 3, 4, 2

ⓔ 3, 4, 5

37. Which one of the following instruments used in the slow-speed handpiece functions to spin filling materials into root canals?

ⓐ Gates-Glidden bur

ⓑ Peeso reamer

ⓒ reamer with lateral attachment

ⓓ lentulo spiral

38. The sizes of Gates-Glidden burs are identified by

ⓐ bur length

ⓑ bur diameter

ⓒ shank grooves

ⓓ shank color

39. Using a working length film, endodontic files are measured to the estimated working length, which is how much more or less than the actual measurement from reference point to apex?

ⓐ + 2 mm

ⓑ − 2 mm

ⓒ + 3 mm

ⓓ − 3 mm

40. Numbers 8 or 10 files should NOT be used when taking working length radiographs because

(a) they bind before reaching the apical area

(b) their small tips may not be visible on the film

(c) their magnification factor is unknown

(d) they often extend beyond the radiographic apex

41. Endodontic broaches are primarily used for

(a) gross removal of soft tissue from the canal spaces of vital teeth

(b) shaping root canals

(c) enlarging root canals

(d) planing intracanal walls

42. The Gates-Glidden file and the Peeso reamer differ in that the Gates-Glidden file

(a) may or may not have a noncutting safe tip

(b) is engine driven

(c) has an elliptical shape

(d) facilitates opening the canal space

43. An endodontic explorer may be used for

(a) holding gutta percha cones during heat transmission

(b) condensing gutta percha

(c) checking intracanal walls

(d) locating canal orifices

44. Endodontic finger spreaders and pluggers differ in that pluggers

(a) are flat at the end

(b) are used to obturate the canal

(c) may be handled or finger type

(d) are of stainless steel that has not been annealed

45. Trial cones should be no shorter than what distance from the prepared canal length?

(a) 2.5 mm

(b) 2 to 2.5 mm

(c) 1.5 to 2 mm

(d) 1 to 1.5 mm

46. If a root canal master cone appears buckled on a radiograph, it is
    (a) too long
    (b) too short
    (c) too thick
    (d) too small

47. Root canal filling material extruded into the periapical tissue may indicate what procedure?
    (a) apicoectomy
    (b) periapical curettage
    (c) pulpectomy
    (d) pulpotomy

48. In what procedure is a Messing root canal gun used?
    (a) periapical curettage
    (b) vital pulpotomy
    (c) retrofilling
    (d) final filling of root canals

49. The material used in retrofilling is
    (a) zinc oxide – eugenol
    (b) calcium hydroxide
    (c) gutta percha
    (d) zinc-free silver alloy

50. Which of the following forms of illicit drug use could cause a human immunodeficiency virus (HIV)-seropositive test?
    (1) oral
    (2) inhalation
    (3) parenteral
    (4) nonparenteral
        (a) 1, 3
        (b) 2, 4
        (c) 3 only
        (d) 4 only

51. Match the following definitions with the terms that they describe.

① antiseptic _____
② asepsis _____
③ cidal agents _____
④ cross-contamination _____
⑤ disinfection _____
⑥ bioburden _____

ⓐ destruction of most microorganisms
ⓑ freedom from infective microorganisms
ⓒ passage of microorganisms from one person to another
ⓓ a chemical agent applied to inanimate surfaces
ⓔ a chemical agent that may be applied to living tissues to destroy or inhibit microorganisms
ⓕ chemicals that kill microorganisms by irreversible action
ⓖ passage of infection from one person or inanimate object to another
ⓗ the level of organisms on a particular item at a specific time

52. Match the following definitions with the terms that they describe.

① cold sterilant _____
② sanitize _____
③ septic _____
④ sterilization _____

ⓐ unsterile; having infection caused by introduction of pathogenic microorganisms that are highly resistant
ⓑ an agent that sterilizes at room temperature
ⓒ to make an item surgically clean but not necessarily sterile
ⓓ total destruction of all microbial life

53. Which of the following precautions for infection control are considered unnecessary except when a patient is thought to pose a high risk?

① wear masks, gloves, and eye protection
② thoroughly clean all equipment after the patient's dismissal
③ disinfect all operatory surfaces
④ sterilize all instruments
⑤ maintain a sterile treatment area
⑥ practice immunologic protection

    ⓐ 1 only
    ⓑ 1, 3, 4
    ⓒ all of the above
    ⓓ none of the above

54. The Occupational Safety and Health Administration Act (OSHA) requires that

   ① confidential medical records be kept for all employees at the risk of blood-borne pathogen transmission in an occupational setting

   ② all dental patients be treated as though they are HIV and hepatitis B virus (HBV) infected

   ③ extra control barriers that surpass universal precautions be used when providing treatment for a patient who is HIV seropositive

   ④ employers provide HBV vaccine at no charge to their employees who are at risk for HBV infection

      ⓐ 1, 2, 3

      ⓑ 1, 2, 4

      ⓒ 1, 3, 4

      ⓓ 2, 3, 4

      ⓔ 3, 4

55. Which of the following is NOT always true of ultrasonic cleaning?

      ⓐ all particulate is removed

      ⓑ it is more efficient than hand scrubbing

      ⓒ it reduces aerosolization of potentially pathogenic organisms during the cleaning procedure

      ⓓ it reduces the potential for puncture wounds

56. The characteristic that surface disinfectants such as diluted iodophors, synthetic phenols, and chlorines have in common is that they

      ⓐ produce surface asepsis

      ⓑ kill poliovirus

      ⓒ negate the need for ultrasonic cleaners

      ⓓ are good cleaners

57. According to OSHA, employers of workers who might come in contact with blood are responsible for which of the following?

   ① a written "exposure central plan"

   ② providing free hepatitis vaccinations for workers

   ③ providing gloves, masks, and smocks

   ④ identifying workers who might be at risk

   ⑤ ensuring an aseptic working area

      ⓐ 1, 2, 4

      ⓑ 2, 4, 5

      ⓒ 1, 2, 3, 4

ⓓ 2, 3, 4, 5

ⓔ all of the above

58. OSHA guidelines classify tasks into categories according to the risk factor. Under what categories would dental office employees be placed?

① I
② II
③ III
④ IV

ⓐ 1, 2
ⓑ 1, 3
ⓒ 2, 4
ⓓ 1, 2, 3
ⓔ 1, 3, 4

59. Which of the following materials would NOT be used as a protective barrier on the head of an x-ray machine?

ⓐ foil
ⓑ plastic wrap
ⓒ disposable paper cover
ⓓ washable cloth cover

60. Match the required sterilization information with the form of sterilization listed.

① dry heat _____
② chemical vapor _____
③ autoclave _____
④ flash _____

ⓐ 15 psi at 121°C for 20 to 40 minutes
ⓑ 160°C for 120 minutes or 170°C for 60 minutes
ⓒ 30 psi at 132°C for 3 to 8 minutes
ⓓ 20 to 40 psi at 132°C for 20 minutes
ⓔ 10 psi at 160°C for 10 minutes
ⓕ 112°C for 60 minutes or 212°C for 30 minutes

61. Three of the more common problems related to diminished efficiency of office sterilization procedures are

① operator error
② improper wrapping of instruments
③ unstable solutions
④ defective control gauges

Continued on next page

(a) 1, 2, 3

(b) 1, 2, 4

(c) 1, 3, 4

(d) 2, 3, 4

62. The merit in the use of holding solutions is that they

① preclude the need for ultrasonic cleaning

② begin microbial kill on soiled instruments

③ prevent air-borne transmission of dried microorganisms

④ minimize handling of soiled instruments

⑤ prevent debris from drying on instruments

    (a) 1, 2, 3, 5

    (b) 1, 2, 4, 5

    (c) 1, 2, 3, 4

    (d) 2, 3, 4, 5

63. The problem existing when the exterior surfaces of handpieces are cleaned and then exposed to disinfectants for 10 minutes is that

    (a) because of the time involved in the procedure, excessive numbers of handpieces must be purchased

    (b) surface disinfectant remaining on the handpiece may be irritating to a patient's oral tissues

    (c) the interior portion of the handpiece is not disinfected

    (d) surface disinfectants eventually cause staining and pitting of handpieces

64. Which of the following is true in regard to the use of disposable face masks?

① disposable face masks are next in importance to disposable gloves

② they make it more difficult to transmit oral pathogens than nasal ones

③ the accepted minimum requirement of face masks is 95 percent filtration of particles 3 to 5 microns in size

④ their use under a shield is recommended to prevent transmission of respiratory pathogens

⑤ they are primarily used to cover the nasal mucosa

    (a) 1, 2, 3, 4

    (b) 1, 3, 5

    (c) 1, 4, 5

    (d) 2, 3, 4

    (e) all of the above

65. By using the letters next to the list of disinfectant solutions, indicate which may be recommended for the following impressions. The letters may be used once, more than once, or not at all.

① alginate _____   ⓐ glutaraldehydes

② polysulfide rubber base _____   ⓑ iodophors

③ silicone rubber _____   ⓒ chlorine compounds

④ polyether _____   ⓓ complex phenolics

⑤ zinc oxide–eugenol impression paste _____   ⓔ phenolic glutaraldehydes

⑥ reversible hydrocolloid _____

⑦ compound _____

66. Which of the following applies to infection control for partial or complete removable dentures in the dental laboratory?

① disinfect new prostheses after their construction

② rag polishing wheels are discarded, laundered, or autoclaved after each use

③ fresh pumice is used for polishing each dental prosthesis

④ place finished prostheses in moist, sealed bags

     ⓐ 1, 2, 3

     ⓑ 2, 3, 4

     ⓒ 3, 4

     ⓓ all of the above

67. Using the following schematic drawing, label the injection sites by matching the letters to the numbered descriptions.

① infraorbital _____

② nasopalatine _____

③ long buccal _____

④ mental _____

⑤ greater palatine _____

⑥ mandibular nerve block _____

⑦ maxillary molars _____

(From Torres H, Ehrlich A: Modern Dental Assisting, 4th ed. Philadelphia, WB Saunders, 1990, p 185)

68. Capping the needle of a used anesthetic syringe is accomplished by

    (a) holding the needle guard (cap) in one hand and the syringe in the other hand

    (b) placing the needle guard on a tray and placing the needle into a needle guard

    (c) slipping a guard over the needle while holding the needle

    (d) placing a needle guard on the syringe held by the operator

69. The syringe needle used for a mandibular block injection should be what length and gauge?

    (a) 32 gauge and 3/4 inch long

    (b) 30 gauge and 1 inch long

    (c) 27 gauge and 1 1/4 inches long

    (d) 25 gauge and 1 5/8 inches long

70. In intraosseous anesthesia, the operator deposits the local anesthetic solution

    (1) through the oral mucosa

    (2) through the cortical plate of the alveolus

    (3) into the cancellous portion of the alveolus

    (a) 1 only

    (b) 3 only

    (c) 2, 3

    (d) 1, 2, 3

71. Which of the following local anesthetics may be selected for a patient with a history of heart disease, hyperthyroidism, or hypertension?

    (1) solution without epinephrine

    (2) solution without neo-Cobefrin

    (3) solution with neo-Cobefrin

    (4) solution with epinephrine

    (a) 1, 2

    (b) 1, 3

    (c) 2, 4

    (d) 4 only

72. The accepted procedure when handling a loaded syringe is to

    (1) recap the needle cautiously after a check of solution from the syringe

    (2) place the ring of the syringe on the operator's thumb

③ turn the lumen (bevel) of the needle toward the alveolus

④ turn the lumen (bevel) of the needle toward the hard palate

    ⓐ 1, 3

    ⓑ 2, 4

    ⓒ 1, 2, 3

    ⓓ 4 only

73. After loading the syringe with a Carpule of local anesthetic solution, the assistant should

  ① retract the plunger to locate the harpoon

  ② firmly tap the ring or base of the syringe attaching the harpoon to the rubber plunger

  ③ draw the plunger backward to ensure attachment of the harpoon

  ④ expel droplets of anesthetic solution to determine an open syringe needle

  ⑤ cautiously replace the needle cover

    ⓐ 1, 3

    ⓑ 2, 4

    ⓒ 2, 3, 4, 5

    ⓓ all of the above

74. Infiltration anesthesia of the dental tissues is produced by chemical reaction on the

    ⓐ facial nerve trunk

    ⓑ anterior branch of the trigeminal nerve

    ⓒ posterior branch of the trigeminal nerve

    ⓓ plexus of the branches of the trigeminal nerve

75. Vasoconstrictor materials are added to an anesthetic solution to

  ① restrict circulation of blood in the tissues at the site of the injection

  ② retain the action of the anesthesia in the tissues

  ③ decrease blood loss during oral surgery

  ④ stimulate circulation of blood in the tissues

    ⓐ 1, 3

    ⓑ 2, 4

    ⓒ 1, 2, 3

    ⓓ 2, 3, 4

76. Topical anesthetic ointment is swabbed on the oral mucosa at the site of the injection to

① desensitize the mucosa
② prevent infection after the injection
③ serve as a palliative agent
④ serve as an antiseptic agent

ⓐ 1, 3
ⓑ 2, 4
ⓒ 1, 2, 3
ⓓ 4 only

77. Which of the following is necessary at the time a patient is to be administered general anesthesia?

① an update of the complete medical history
② an anesthetist as a member of the team
③ an evaluation of medical history and potential patient risk
④ review of presurgical instructions with the patient

ⓐ 1, 3
ⓑ 2, 4
ⓒ 1, 2, 3
ⓓ all of the above

78. Which of the following may cause the condition of paresthesia?

① injection of contaminated anesthetic solution
② trauma to a nerve sheath
③ hemorrhaging in or around the nerve sheath
④ excessive amount of anesthetic solution injected

ⓐ 1, 3
ⓑ 2, 4
ⓒ 1, 2, 3
ⓓ 4 only

79. The planes of analgesia generally considered safe for use in dentistry are

① Plane I
② Plane II
③ Plane III
④ Plane IV

(a) 1, 2

(b) 3, 4

(c) 1, 2, 3

(d) all of the above

80. During the administration of nitrous oxide–oxygen analgesia, a patient's base-line is characterized by

① comfort and cooperation

② intact and active reflexes

③ normal vital signs

④ hyperactivity

(a) 1, 3

(b) 2, 4

(c) 1, 2, 3

(d) 4 only

81. On which of the following anatomic sites is anesthetic solution placed to anesthetize the maxillary central incisors?

(a) the mucogingival junction of the apices and the facial mucosa

(b) inferior alveolar foramen

(c) maxillary incisive papilla

(d) mental foramen

82. Which of the following instrumentation is used to effect local anesthesia of the mandibular first molar (tooth #19)?

① topical anesthetic on the mucosa, at the left inferior alveolar foramen

② topical anesthetic on the mucosa, at the right inferior alveolar foramen

③ local anesthetic with an aspirating syringe and 27-gauge needle

④ local anesthetic with an aspirating syringe and 18-gauge needle

(a) 1, 3

(b) 2, 3

(c) 1, 4

(d) 2, 4

83. When preparing and passing a local anesthetic syringe to the dentist for anesthesia of tooth #29, the assistant

① prepares an aspirating syringe with a Carpule of local anesthetic and a 28-gauge needle

Continued on next page

② swabs the lingual area of the left mandibular mucosa near the inferior mandibular foramen

③ passes an aspirating syringe, placing the ring on the operator's thumb

④ uncaps the cover from the needle and turns the lumen (bevel) toward the mucosa

    ⓐ 1, 3

    ⓑ 2, 4

    ⓒ 1, 3, 4

    ⓓ 2, 3, 4

84. When using the infiltration technique, which of the following agents would produce fast-acting local anesthesia for intermediate duration?

    ⓐ Carbocaine (mepivacaine hydrochloride USP) without a vasoconstrictor

    ⓑ Carbocaine (mepivacaine hydrochloride 2 percent/neo-Cobefrin 1:20,000)

    ⓒ Ravocaine (hydrochloride 0.4 percent, Novocain 2 percent, neo-Cobefrin 1:20,000)

    ⓓ Marcaine (bupivacaine hydrochloride 0.50 percent with epinephrine 1:200,000)

85. Which of the following meet the criteria for topical anesthetic material?

① effective on the oral mucosa

② suppression of gag reflex

③ onset within 4 to 6 seconds

④ allergic reaction rare

    ⓐ 1, 3

    ⓑ 2, 4

    ⓒ 1, 2, 4

    ⓓ 2, 3, 4

86. Tuberculosis, herpes, acquired immunodeficiency syndrome, and hepatitis B have in common the fact that they

    ⓐ are sexually transmitted

    ⓑ may be spread by contaminated food or water

    ⓒ may be transmitted by a carrier

    ⓓ are first manifested in the oral cavity

87. When a patient demonstrates symptoms of diabetic acidosis, staff members should

(a) inject the patient with insulin

(b) place a sugar cube under the patient's tongue

(c) seek medical aid

(d) advise the patient to contact his or her physician

88. The body's initial inflammatory response to injury is

① a primary internal defense mechanism

② protective in character

③ the cause of necrosis

④ undesirable in that it curtails the body's immune system

(a) 1, 2

(b) 1, 3, 4

(c) 2, 3

(d) 2, 4

89. The carotid pulse may be found in the area of the

(a) larynx

(b) pharynx

(c) clavicle

(d) parotid gland

(e) a, c

90. During cardiopulmonary resuscitation (CPR) on an adult, if the head is in the correct position and the airway is blocked, the next step is to

① place the patient in a supine position

② position the patient so that a firm thump can be administered to the back

③ use a finger to sweep the oral cavity

④ begin compressing the sternum

⑤ perform the abdominal thrust

(a) 1, 3

(b) 2, 4

(c) 3, 4

(d) 3, 5

91. Which of the following are true when two rescuers are applying CPR to an adult?

① the rate of compression is 80 to 100 compressions per minute

② the patient is ventilated on the downstroke

Continued on next page

③ the rate is five compressions to one lung inflation

④ the depth of compression is 1 1/2 to 2 inches

    ⓐ 1, 2, 3

    ⓑ 1, 3, 4

    ⓒ 1, 4

    ⓓ 2, 3, 4

92. Symptoms of anaphylactic shock include

① edema

② urticaria

③ convulsions

④ cyanosis

⑤ bradycardia

    ⓐ 1, 2, 3

    ⓑ 1, 2, 4

    ⓒ 1, 4, 5

    ⓓ 2, 3, 4

    ⓔ all of the above

93. Treatment for the condition of postural hypoxemia may include

    ⓐ forcing patients to consume liquids

    ⓑ positioning patients in a supine position

    ⓒ ingestion of carbohydrates by patient

    ⓓ slowly positioning patients upright

94. First aid for obstruction of an adult patient's airway by a foreign object may include

① injection of a muscle relaxant

② nothing if the patient is coughing or can speak

③ closed chest massage

④ a finger sweep of the oropharynx to dislodge the object

    ⓐ 1, 3

    ⓑ 2 only

    ⓒ 1, 3

    ⓓ 4 only

95. The symptoms of an angina pectoris attack include
    ① flushed skin
    ② substernal pain
    ③ erythema
    ④ cyanosis
       ⓐ 1, 3
       ⓑ 2, 4
       ⓒ 1, 2, 3
       ⓓ 4 only

96. The first aid procedures for patients suffering an attack of angina pectoris include
    ① placing them in a supine position
    ② seating them upright
    ③ administering 100 percent oxygen
    ④ administering one nitroglycerin tablet sublingually
       ⓐ 1, 4
       ⓑ 2, 3
       ⓒ 1, 3, 4
       ⓓ 2, 3, 4

97. If pulmonary arrest is evident (adult patient), a rescuer places the heel of one open hand (intertwined with the other hand)
    ⓐ on the midline of the sternum
    ⓑ immediately below the xiphoid
    ⓒ on the diaphragm
    ⓓ about two fingers' width above the tip of the xiphoid

98. Diabetic acidosis may be brought on if a diabetic patient has
    ① failed to take medication on fixed schedule
    ② eaten too much sweet food
    ③ failed to eat on a fixed schedule
    ④ has an infection
       ⓐ 1, 3
       ⓑ 2, 4
       ⓒ 1, 2, 3
       ⓓ all of the above

99. What should be done for conscious patients showing symptoms of insulin shock (hypoglycemic shock)?

- ⓐ give refined carbohydrates
- ⓑ withhold refined carbohydrates
- ⓒ advise patients to increase insulin intake
- ⓓ advise patients to rest without eating

100. A Class III injury to a tooth crown involves

- ⓐ fracture of the incisal margin of the enamel
- ⓑ mesioincisal fracture of the enamel
- ⓒ fracture of the crown, exposing the pulp
- ⓓ traumatization of a tooth, rendering it nonvital

101. Before first aid measures, an assessment of an unconscious victim's condition must determine

- ① if pupils of the eyes contract with light
- ② if the airway is open
- ③ if breathing has ceased
- ④ if a pulse is absent
    - ⓐ 1, 3
    - ⓑ 2, 4
    - ⓒ 2, 3, 4
    - ⓓ 4 only

102. Retraction cord is removed from the gingival sulcus immediately before placing the

- ⓐ second coating of adhesive in the custom tray
- ⓑ tray impression material into the custom tray
- ⓒ syringe-type impression material into the gingival sulcus
- ⓓ tray loaded with putty material onto the teeth in the quadrant

103. The advantage of visible light-cured types of impression materials is that they

- ① provide longer working time
- ② set faster
- ③ polymerize when exposed to ultraviolet light
- ④ produce more detailed impressions
    - ⓐ 1, 3
    - ⓑ 2, 3

© 2, 4

@ 4 only

104. Which of the following materials may be placed into an ill-fitting denture to relieve irritation of underlying tissues?

① temporary soft reliners

② tissue conditioners

③ plasticized acrylic resins

④ zinc oxide – eugenol paste

   ⓐ 1, 3

   ⓑ 2, 4

   ⓒ 1, 2, 3

   ⓓ 3, 4

105. Which of the following provides even space for impression material when fabricating a custom tray?

① lubricating the cast with a separating medium

② reducing the base plate wax 2 mm from the finish line of the tray

③ warming the impression tray before placing base plate wax

④ placing two layers of the base plate wax over the cast

   ⓐ 1, 3

   ⓑ 2, 4

   ⓒ 1, 2, 3

   ⓓ 4 only

106. It is necessary to coat custom trays with adhesive before placement of what type of impression material?

① vinyl polysiloxane

② alginates

③ polysulfides

④ polyethers

⑤ hydrocolloids

   ⓐ 1, 3

   ⓑ 2, 4

   ⓒ 1, 3, 4

   ⓓ 5 only

107. When dental supplies are received, they are often accompanied by an itemized list of the supplies sent and their cost. This list is called

    ⓐ a packing slip
    ⓑ an invoice
    ⓒ a statement
    ⓓ a purchase order

108. In order to cash a check, it must be endorsed by the

    ⓐ payor
    ⓑ dentist
    ⓒ payee
    ⓓ bearer

109. When balancing the checkbook with the bank statement, deposits in transit are

    ⓐ subtracted from the bank statement
    ⓑ added to the bank statement
    ⓒ subtracted from the check register
    ⓓ added to the check register

110. Jane Doe receives $1,500 per month, which is paid in two equal installments. Her income tax deduction is 20 percent of her gross pay and her FICA contribution is 8 percent of her gross pay. What is Jane's pay for each pay period?

    ⓐ $490
    ⓑ $510
    ⓒ $540
    ⓓ $575

111. In the problem described in the previous question, what is the employer's contribution for Jane each quarter?

    ⓐ $345
    ⓑ $360
    ⓒ $375
    ⓓ $385

112. In the problem described in question 110, what is the total withholding tax that must be remitted for Jane by the employer at the end of each quarter?

    ⓐ $300
    ⓑ $600

(c) $750

(d) $900

113. The Uniform Code in Dental Procedures and Nomenclature was developed to
    (a) serve as a master file system
    (b) simplify computerized bookkeeping systems
    (c) help coordinate the benefits for patients with dual coverage
    (d) simplify the reporting of dental procedures on insurance forms

114. What is the alloy of choice when difficulty exists in keeping the region dry when placing a silver amalgam restoration?
    (a) mercury free
    (b) zinc free
    (c) tin free
    (d) copper free

115. The custom matrix for a Class II (two or three surface) amalgam restoration may be secured by the use of
    ① carding wax
    ② self-polymerizing acrylic
    ③ stick compound
    ④ a custom wedge
        (a) 1, 3
        (b) 2, 4
        (c) 1, 2, 3
        (d) 4 only

116. The procedure for removing a wedge and matrix after condensation and carving of an amalgam restoration includes
    ① using a hemostat to remove the wedge from the lingual aspect
    ② loosening the retainer and removing the wedge from the occlusal aspect
    ③ using cotton pliers to carefully turn ends of the band away from fresh amalgam
    ④ easing the band in an angular direction away from the fresh amalgam
    ⑤ loosening the retainer and lifting the band straight toward the occlusal aspect
        (a) 1, 3
        (b) 2, 4

Continued on next page

(c) 1, 3, 4, 5

(d) 2, 3, 4, 5

117. Armamentarium for placing, condensing, and carving a Class V amalgam restoration includes

① serrated and smooth condensers

② commercial matrix and retainer

③ interproximal carvers

④ Hollenback carver

(a) 1, 3

(b) 1, 4

(c) 2, 3

(d) 2, 4

118. The criteria for acceptability when placing a Tofflemire matrix and wedge include

① the retainer is parallel to the facial surface of the tooth

② the band is trimmed to within 1 mm above the occlusal margin of the tooth

③ the wedge is always placed from the facial aspect at the widest opening of the gingival embrasure

④ the flat surface of the wedge is inserted away from the gingiva

(a) 1, 2

(b) 1, 3

(c) 2, 4

(d) 3, 4

119. Implants should engage cortical bone because

(a) it is spongy and so provides for movement during mastication

(b) location and density of cortical bone are usually constant

(c) trabecular bone is often NOT present in a selected anatomic zone

(d) cortical bone provides for a wider ridge

120. Implants are contraindicated for patients who

① are immunocompromised

② are calcium deficient

③ have insulin-dependent diabetes

④ have hypertension

⑤ are abusers of drugs

(a) 1, 2, 4

(b) 1, 3, 4

(c) 1, 2, 3, 5

(d) 2, 4, 5

121. Implants are classified into categories by their relation to bone. Match the categories with their placement.

① endosseous _____   (a) on bone

② transosseous _____   (b) in bone

③ subperiosteal _____   (c) under bone

                          (d) through bone

122. In cases of peri-implantitis, the specialist who would be responsible for providing comprehensive therapy and establishing effective maintenance is

(a) an oral surgeon

(b) an endodontist

(c) a prosthodontist

(d) a periodontist

123. The routine use of antimicrobials, such as chlorhexidine, as a part of peri-implant home care have been advocated to

(a) prevent calculus build-up

(b) control plaque accumulation

(c) aid in tissue regeneration

(d) disinfect pockets

124. For scaling around implants, the setup should include instruments that are

① Teflon

② plastic

③ wooden

④ metal

⑤ gold tipped

(a) 1, 2, 3

(b) 1, 2, 4

(c) 1, 2, 3, 5

(d) 1, 3, 4, 5

125. Which of the following may be used for effective implant home care?

    ① hard brushes

    ② cuttlefish polishing strips

    ③ yarn

    ④ end-tufted brushes

    ⑤ oral irrigators

        ⓐ 1, 2, 3

        ⓑ 1, 3, 4

        ⓒ 2, 3, 5

        ⓓ 3, 4, 5

126. When an operator is preparing the buccal surface of a mandibular molar, an assistant may place the aspirator tip

    ① on the buccal surface mesial to the handpiece

    ② on the buccal surface distal to the handpiece

    ③ in a position to retract the cheek

    ④ lingual to the molar

        ⓐ 1, 3

        ⓑ 2 only

        ⓒ 2, 3

        ⓓ 3 only

127. The depth placement of a dowel post used to support a crown on a nonvital tooth should be

    ⓐ the same as the overall length of the crown

    ⓑ two times the depth of the crown

    ⓒ one-half the overall length of the unprepared tooth

    ⓓ two times the length of the gutta percha placed toward the apex

128. Keyway slots function to

    ⓐ form a retention for the crown

    ⓑ prevent loosening of the dowel post

    ⓒ form retention for core build-ups

    ⓓ ensure that pin holes are parallel to the path of insertion of the finished crown

129. Which of the following sequences is correct for obtaining a paste bite registration?

① place utility wax on the loop of the bite frame

② extrude the accelerator and base onto the pad

③ insert gauze onto the bite frame opposite the wax

④ place the bulk of the mixture on the maxillary side of the gauze

⑤ draw a gauze bib over the wax and affix it

⑥ place the cross-wire of the frame mesial to the posterior mandibular teeth

⑦ trim the excess gauze

⑧ remove the bit frame and impression after about 3 minutes

    (a) 1, 3, 5, 7, 4, 6, 8

    (b) 1, 3, 5, 7, 2, 8

    (c) 1, 3, 5, 7, 6, 8

    (d) 1, 3, 5, 2, 4, 6, 8

130. Temporary crowns on posterior teeth must

① contact adjacent teeth

② have a minimum of three contacts with opposing teeth

③ have sealed margins

④ have trim lines remaining as scribed

    (a) 1, 2

    (b) 1, 3

    (c) 2, 3

    (d) all of the above

131. When constructing a custom tray using the vacuum technique, the material used to form a space is

    (a) wax

    (b) acrylic

    (c) Styrofoam

    (d) aluminum foil

132. Match the units of a removable partial with their function by placing the appropriate letter in the blank.

① stress breaker _____
② framework _____
③ saddle _____
④ bar _____
⑤ clasp _____
⑥ rest _____

ⓐ a piece of metal serving as a connector
ⓑ a metal skeleton
ⓒ retains the artificial teeth
ⓓ helps to support and provide stability to the partial denture
ⓔ controls the extent of seating of the prosthesis
ⓕ relieves the abutment teeth of excessive occlusal loads

133. In addition to registering the occlusal relationship of the two dental arches, occlusal bite rims register

ⓐ lateral dimension
ⓑ mesiodistal dimension
ⓒ vertical dimension
ⓓ lateral excursion

134. A prosthesis seated on a partially edentulous arch in which the teeth have been prepared with copings is

ⓐ a partial denture
ⓑ a template
ⓒ an overdenture
ⓓ a duplicate denture

135. Vent plant implants function to

ⓐ improve stability
ⓑ encourage alveolus regeneration
ⓒ provide support to mandibular prostheses
ⓓ stabilize abutments for removable prostheses

136. Which one of the following teeth is most likely to suffer furcation involvement?

ⓐ maxillary second premolar
ⓑ maxillary second molar
ⓒ mandibular canine
ⓓ mandibular second premolar

137. Removal of microbial plaque leads to

    (a) attainment and/or preservation of oral health

    (b) resolution of gingival recession

    (c) retardation of systemic factors related to development of periodontal disease

    (d) resolution of decalcification

138. Which of the following is true in regard to plaque removal?

    (a) three to four cleanings a day produce significantly better periodontal conditions

    (b) emphasis should be placed on efficiency rather than frequency of cleaning

    (c) plaque may be controlled by efficient brushing

    (d) a professional polishing at 3-month intervals is sufficient to maintain a healthy oral environment

139. Clinical changes that should be recognized in cases of chronic gingivitis include

    ① sloughing and grayish particles

    ② soggy puffiness that pits on pressure

    ③ vesicle formation

    ④ pinpoint surface areas of redness and desquamation

        (a) 1, 2

        (b) 1, 3

        (c) 2, 3

        (d) 2, 4

140. Characteristic clinical signs of acute necrotizing ulcerative gingivitis include

    ① spontaneous gingival hemorrhage

    ② punched-out interdental papillae

    ③ decreased salivation

    ④ fetid odor

    ⑤ slow onset

        (a) 1, 2, 3

        (b) 1, 2, 4

        (c) 2, 3, 5

        (d) 2, 4, 5

141. Factors predisposing to acute necrotizing ulcerative gingivitis include

① smoking
② direct communication
③ pre-existing chronic gingival disease
④ antibiotic therapy

ⓐ 1, 2
ⓑ 1, 3
ⓒ 1, 4
ⓓ 2, 4

142. Place the letter best describing a form of gingivitis in the blank next to the type listed.

① localized gingivitis _____
② localized marginal gingivitis _____
③ diffuse gingivitis _____
④ generalized diffuse gingivitis _____

ⓐ involves the gingival margin, attached gingiva, and interdental papillae
ⓑ confined to the gingival margins of a single tooth or a group of teeth
ⓒ involves the gingival margin in relation to all the teeth as well as the interdental papillae
ⓓ confined to one or more areas of the gingival margin
ⓔ involves the entire gingiva, usually affecting the alveolar mucosa

143. Which of the following features characterize a suprabony periodontal pocket?

① the base of the pocket is apical to the crest of the alveolar bone
② the bone destructive pattern is vertically angular
③ the pattern of the bone is horizontal
④ the base of the pocket is coronal to the level of the alveolar bone

ⓐ 1, 2
ⓑ 1, 3
ⓒ 2, 4
ⓓ 3, 4

144. A periodontal pack should be applied

① to cover the incised gingival margin
② first to the facial aspect
③ first to the lingual area

④ to extend to the occlusal or incisal surface

⑤ to extend interproximally

    ⓐ 1, 2, 4

    ⓑ 1, 2, 5

    ⓒ 1, 4, 5

    ⓓ 3, 4, 5

145. Information given to a patient suffering from root sensitivity after periodontal treatment should include what two facts?

① desensitizing agents should provide immediate relief

② desensitizing agents may be applied in the dental office or by the patient when at home

③ plaque control is important in reducing sensitivity

④ plaque control efforts may be eliminated until resolution of sensitivity

    ⓐ 1, 2

    ⓑ 1, 3

    ⓒ 2, 3

    ⓓ 2, 4

146. In addition to being a reliable clinical tool for identifying pockets, a periodontal probe is used to

① measure gingival recession

② identify caries

③ locate calculus

④ resolve bleeding

⑤ remove calculus

⑥ determine mucobuccal relationships

    ⓐ 1, 2, 3

    ⓑ 1, 2, 4

    ⓒ 1, 3, 5

    ⓓ 1, 3, 6

    ⓔ 1, 5, 6

147. Which of the following are true in regard to techniques used to probe a complete dentition?

① the mouth is considered in sextants

② the first tooth to be probed is the maxillary right central incisor

③ six probing depth measurements are taken on each tooth

Continued on next page

④ the technique precisely measures the depths of the anatomic structures

⑤ the deepest measurement on each surface is recorded

ⓐ 1, 2, 4

ⓑ 1, 3, 5

ⓒ 1, 4, 5

ⓓ 2, 3, 5

148. The use of an ultrasonic scaler is NOT contraindicated in a patient with

ⓐ a cardiac pacemaker

ⓑ an infectious disease

ⓒ Class II and Class III furcation lesions

ⓓ resin restorations

149. Morse scalers are included on the tray of scaling and root planing instruments for use in

ⓐ long narrow pockets in the region of thin roots

ⓑ removing supragingival calculus in the contact areas of anterior teeth

ⓒ removing gross calculus in subgingival areas

ⓓ root planing

150. When charting tooth mobility, the number used to indicate total movement of 1 mm displacement is

ⓐ 0

ⓑ 1

ⓒ 2

ⓓ 3

151. Coronal polishing is indicated for

① removing extrinsic stains

② applying a rubber dam

③ disclosure of decalcified areas

④ caries prevention

ⓐ 1, 2

ⓑ 3, 4

ⓒ 1, 4

ⓓ 2, 3

152. All of the following are reasons for polishing teeth with an abrasive agent after scaling EXCEPT to

(a) remove plaque

(b) render a smooth tooth surface

(c) remove stains resulting from poor oral hygiene

(d) remove intrinsic stains

153. Under what circumstances is a porte polisher used during a coronal polishing procedure?

(1) when the creation of aerosol is considered to be particularly hazardous

(2) when teeth are extremely sensitive to heat

(3) when stain is particularly heavy

(4) when several teeth are missing in an arch

(a) 1, 2

(b) 2, 3

(c) 2, 4

(d) 3, 4

154. A normal sulcus depth is

(a) 6 mm

(b) 4 mm

(c) 3 mm

(d) 2 mm

155. By placing check marks in the blanks, indicate the proper tray setup for periodontal examination and charting.

(a) basic setup ____

(b) set of Gracey scalers ____

(c) porte polisher ____

(d) periodontal probe ____

(e) cotton pellets ____

(f) mandrel and cuttlefish disks ____

(g) sterile gauze squares ____

(h) dental floss ____

(i) tooth mobility detector ____

(j) high-velocity evacuation tip ____

(k) periodontal chart ____

(l) red and blue pencils ____

156. Fluorides act to prevent dental caries by all of the following mechanisms EXCEPT

(a) increasing the resistance of tooth structure to acid dissolution

(b) enhancing the process of remineralization

(c) neutralizing the pH of plaque formations

(d) reducing the cariogenic potential of dental plaque

157. The use of calcium hydroxide in primary teeth may be contraindicated because it

(a) frequently stimulates internal resorption

(b) often produces acute pulpal inflammation

(c) may stimulate calcific formations

(d) frequently contributes to ankylosis

158. Which of the following is an indication for sealant placement?

(a) well-coalesced self-cleansing fissures

(b) stained fissures

(c) pits and fissures appearing to be decalcified

(d) deep retentive pits and fissures in which an explorer may catch

159. Before extraction, a tooth is luxated in order to

(a) loosen the periosteum

(b) free the roots

(c) compress the bone and enlarge the socket

(d) make sure it is not ankylosed

160. Which one of the following procedures would be used to correct a diastema?

(a) alveolectomy

(b) frenectomy

(c) osteotomy

(d) luxation

161. Sutures are cut at what distance beyond the knot?

(a) 0.5 mm

(b) 1 mm

(c) 2 to 3 mm

(d) 4 mm

162. The number of sutures placed is noted on a patient's chart in order to
    ⓐ indicate the extent of the surgery
    ⓑ give support to the fee charged
    ⓒ act as a guide when checking suture absorption
    ⓓ compare with the number of sutures removed

163. An exfoliative cytologic evaluation requires
    ⓐ surgical removal of a portion of the lesion
    ⓑ aspiration of the lesion
    ⓒ scraping of the surface of the lesion
    ⓓ excision of the entire lesion

164. Which classification used in a cytologic report would be suggestive of a malignancy but not conclusive?
    ⓐ II
    ⓑ III
    ⓒ IV
    ⓓ V

165. A periosteotome is used to
    ⓐ pry a tooth from its socket
    ⓑ remove debris from the socket
    ⓒ remove the periodontium from the tooth root
    ⓓ detach the gingival tissue from around the cervix of a tooth

166. Which forms of fat should be recommended to patients trying to decrease their serum cholesterol level?
    ① polyunsaturated
    ② monounsaturated
    ③ saturated
    ④ trans fatty
        ⓐ 1 only
        ⓑ 1, 2
        ⓒ 3, 4
        ⓓ 4 only

167. Which of the following foods would be advised for dental patients with cardiovascular disease?

Continued on next page

① processed cheese and/or canned shrimp
② olives, chicken bouillon, salted cashews
③ any kosher foods
④ pasta, rice, potatoes
⑤ green leafy vegetables
⑥ citrus fruits and bananas
⑦ corn chips, potato chips, onion rings

    ⓐ 1, 2, 3
    ⓑ 3, 5, 6
    ⓒ 4, 5, 6
    ⓓ 3, 5, 7

168. When counseling a patient in regard to diet and caries prevention, which facts should be emphasized?

① the role of dental plaque in caries development
② a description of cariogenic and noncariogenic foods
③ the need for immediate and radical reform of poor dietary habits
④ the relationship of simple carbohydrates to the formation of decay
⑤ the need to abstain permanently from all foods that promote decay

    ⓐ 1, 2
    ⓑ 1, 2, 4
    ⓒ 1, 3, 5
    ⓓ 2, 4, 5

169. Which of the following breakfasts would be suggested for a postextraction patient?

    ⓐ enriched dry toast, fried eggs, low-fat bacon, milk, and half a grapefruit
    ⓑ cooked cereal with milk, applesauce, and milk or juice
    ⓒ buttered whole wheat toast, ham omelet, fresh pear, and milk or juice
    ⓓ dry cereal with milk or cream and sliced banana, slice of buttered whole wheat toast, and two pieces of crisp bacon

170. When counseling dental patients about their diet, consideration must be given to

① cultural background
② food habits
③ knowledge of basic nutrition
④ economic status
⑤ physical condition

     (a) 2, 4

     (b) 2, 4, 5

     (c) 1, 3, 4

     (d) all of the above

171. From the foods listed below, select the nutrients most abundant in each.

     (a) vitamin A

     (b) B vitamins

     (c) vitamin C

     (d) calcium

     (e) protein

     (f) carbohydrates

     (g) iron

  (1) citrus fruit and tomatoes:_____, _____

  (2) broccoli, spinach, carrots, cantaloupes:_____, _____

  (3) milk and cheese:_____, _____

  (4) meats and poultry:_____, _____, _____

172. Which of the following conditions are contraindications to the use of relative analgesia?

  (1) upper respiratory tract infection

  (2) difficulty in communicating with the staff

  (3) advanced emphysema

  (4) emotional instability

     (a) 1, 3

     (b) 2, 4

     (c) 4 only

     (d) all of the above

173. Advantages of relative analgesia may include

  (1) alert and cooperative patient

  (2) rapid and complete recovery when the gases are removed

  (3) ease of administration

  (4) possible use with respiratory problems

     (a) 1, 3

     (b) 2, 4

     (c) 1, 2, 3

     (d) 4 only

174. After the check of the tank's contents and pressure, which of the following are necessary when administering nitrous oxide–oxygen?

① ensure that tank gauges are operating correctly

② the air vent of the patient's mask is closed, and the exhaust valve is open

③ the patient is given 5 to 8 liters of 100 percent oxygen for 1 minute

④ oxygen is reduced 1 liter per minute, nitrous oxide is increased 1 liter per minute

⑤ the patient's baseline values are achieved

   ⓐ 1, 5

   ⓑ 2, 3, 4

   ⓒ 1, 3, 4, 5

   ⓓ all of the above

175. If a patient on nitrous oxide–oxygen is snorting, it means that the

① patient is breathing too deeply

② mask has sealed around the nostrils

③ patient is breathing too lightly

④ patient has reached baseline

   ⓐ 1, 2

   ⓑ 2, 3

   ⓒ 2, 4

   ⓓ 4 only

176. If a patient becomes nauseated when receiving nitrous oxide–oxygen, the assistant immediately

① administers 100 percent oxygen

② turns off the nitrous oxide valve

③ elevates the patient's head

④ increases the amount of nitrous oxide

   ⓐ 1, 2

   ⓑ 1, 3

   ⓒ 3, 4

   ⓓ 1, 2, 3

177. When a dental procedure is concluded and a patient remains anesthetized, how are the valves of the nitrous oxide–oxygen unit adjusted?

① nitrous oxide to 0

② oxygen to 0

③ nitrous oxide to 100

④ oxygen to 100

    ⓐ 1, 2

    ⓑ 1, 4

    ⓒ 2, 3

    ⓓ 2, 4

178. Vinyl polysiloxane impression materials that are supplied in prefilled disposable syringes may be set by

    ⓐ warm air

    ⓑ warm water

    ⓒ visible white light

    ⓓ natural light

179. For each of the lettered setting actions of gypsum materials, match the probable cause. Some of the lettered items have more than one number.

① too much water   ⓐ _____ rapid set

② too little water   ⓑ _____ slow set

③ too rapid, too long spatulation   ⓒ _____ weak set

④ too little spatulation   ⓓ _____ strong set

⑤ cool water

⑥ recommended amount of water

180. Gypsum-bonded investment materials that are refractory have been found to

① expand without fracturing in a burn-out oven

② withstand cold curing on the laboratory bench

③ compensate for the shrinkage that occurs during cooling of casting

④ withstand heating beyond 1,700°F in a burn-out oven

    ⓐ 1, 3

    ⓑ 2 only

    ⓒ 1, 2, 3

    ⓓ 4 only

181. A cast restoration that is prepared to receive a veneer is referred to as a

    ⓐ porcelain-fused-to-metal crown

    ⓑ full cast crown

    ⓒ three-quarters cast crown

    ⓓ full porcelain crown

182. Custom temporary coverage for crown and bridge preparations is constructed of self-polymerizing resins placed in

① reversible hydrocolloid impressions
② primary alginate impressions
③ compound impressions
④ carding wax impressions

ⓐ 1 only
ⓑ 2 only
ⓒ 1, 3
ⓓ 2, 4

183. After cementation of a permanent cast crown, the excess cement is removed

① immediately using an explorer
② by flushing the tooth with copious amounts of water
③ cautiously before final set of cement
④ using a Gracey scaler

ⓐ 1 only
ⓑ 1, 3
ⓒ 2 only
ⓓ 3, 4

184. The mix of zinc phosphate cement for an insulating base is placed in the tooth preparation using

① an explorer
② a spoon excavator
③ a smooth condenser

ⓐ 1 only
ⓑ 3 only
ⓒ 1, 3
ⓓ 2, 3
ⓔ 1, 2, 3

185. The insulating cement base placed in a tooth preparation should cover the pulpal area to a maximum thickness of

ⓐ 1.00 to 1.50 mm
ⓑ 0.75 to 1.00 mm
ⓒ 0.50 to 0.75 mm
ⓓ 0.25 to 0.50 mm

186. Which of the following is NOT true of zinc oxide–eugenol cement?

    (a) mixes quickly to a homogeneous consistency

    (b) is placed over calcium hydroxide on a near pulpal exposure

    (c) is placed over calcium hydroxide in a vital pulpotomy

    (d) is placed over the pulpal area to protect the pulp from thermal shock

    (e) fails to set up in the presence of saliva

187. Which of the following apply when placing a rubber dam over a three-unit fixed bridge?

    ① the anchor tooth punch hole is larger

    ② the anchor tooth punch hole is smaller

    ③ facial and lingual punch holes are made to accommodate the pontic

    ④ abutment teeth are covered

    (a) 1, 3

    (b) 2, 3

    (c) 2, 4

    (d) 4 only

188. The template of a rubber dam punch has how many punch holes to accommodate different sizes of teeth?

    (a) 2

    (b) 3

    (c) 4

    (d) 5

189. In the instrument formula 13-80-8-14, the 80 refers to the

    (a) angle formed by the handle and the blade

    (b) length of the blade

    (c) width of the blade

    (d) angle formed by the cutting edge and the handle

190. If a tooth loses function, the periodontal ligament reacts by

    (a) becoming inflamed

    (b) becoming smaller

    (c) losing sensory capacity

    (d) failing to provide nutrition to the alveolus and cementum

191. Which one of the following is used to stabilize a rubber dam that involves a fixed bridge?
    (a) compound
    (b) wooden wedges
    (c) dental floss or tape
    (d) rubber dam wick

192. The correct position of a Ferrier separator is demonstrated by
    (a) free movement of the separator jaws
    (b) the bows being parallel to the occlusal plane of the teeth
    (c) the amount of tension on the teeth under adjustment
    (d) the position of the separator bolt in relation to adjacent teeth

193. Elliptical burs are characterized by
    (a) round corners and sides
    (b) numerous blades
    (c) elongated shanks
    (d) their use in preparing pin holes in dentin

194. Fiber optics may be provided through
    (a) a mouth mirror
    (b) a traditional operating light
    (c) a high-speed handpiece
    (d) an operator's loupe magnifying glasses

195. Using the letters *a* through *f*, indicate the order of Black's steps for a cavity preparation.
    (a) resistance and retention form _____
    (b) remove carious dentin _____
    (c) refine preparation margins _____
    (d) develop outline form _____
    (e) refine internal portion of cavity _____
    (f) develop access for dentin removal and placement of restoration _____

196. Cotton rolls used to absorb saliva are NOT placed in what area because of its lack of salivary ducts?
    (a) maxillary buccal vestibule
    (b) mandibular buccal vestibule

ⓒ mandibular lingual vestibule

ⓓ maxillary labial vestibule

197. After application, if a rubber dam clamp teeters back and forth, the

ⓐ prongs are too far apart

ⓑ prongs are too close to each other

ⓒ tooth shape is atypical

ⓓ tooth is being securely grasped at its four corners

198. Molar rubber dam applications should usually reach from the first or second molar to the opposite

ⓐ first molar

ⓑ first premolar

ⓒ cuspid

ⓓ lateral

199. When using a Tofflemire retainer, the loop is placed in the right channel when working on which quadrants?

① upper left

② lower left

③ upper right

④ lower right

ⓐ 1, 2

ⓑ 1, 4

ⓒ 2, 3

ⓓ 2, 4

200. Match the following number ranges with the appropriate burs.

① 169 to 171 _____   ⓐ straight fissure, plain cut

② 1/4 to 10 _____   ⓑ inverted cone

③ 55 to 59 _____   ⓒ taper fissure, plain cut

④ 1557 _____   ⓓ round, plain cut

⑤ 33 1/2 to 44 _____   ⓔ straight fissure, cross-cut, round end

⑥ 55 to 560 _____   ⓕ straight fissure cross-cut, dentate

⑦ 699 to 708 _____   ⓖ tapered fissure, cross-cut

201. A large discoid carver is included in an amalgam setup for a restoration

    (a) to refine the anatomy of the filling

    (b) for general shaping

    (c) to begin the groove and fossae formation

    (d) to reduce the area until proper occlusion is achieved

202. Enamel fissures are a result of

    (a) caries activity

    (b) hyperplasia

    (c) failure of lobes to fuse

    (d) fluorosis

203. By using the appropriate numbers, indicate the function of the instruments listed.

    (a) hatchet   ____   (1) cutting

    (b) burnisher   ____   (2) condensing

    (c) Tanner   ____   (3) finishing

    (d) plastic filling ____   (4) carving

    (e) angle formers ____

    (f) discoid-cleoid ____

    (g) file   ____

    (h) knife   ____

204. When an operator is working on a patient's maxillary right facial or occlusal surface, the evacuator tip is placed

    (a) lingual to the handpiece

    (b) facially and mesially to the handpiece

    (c) on the occlusal surface of the mandibular right dentition

    (d) lingual to the mandibular molars

205. Which of the following applies to use of the light-cured systems for light-curable composite resin restorations?

    (1) resin is supplied in a single paste syringe applicator

    (2) resin contains photoinitiator molecules and an amine activator

    (3) the source is usually a fluorescent light bulb

    (4) the tip of the light-curing source is held in contact with the surface resin

    (5) the light-curing source is held for approximately 20 seconds in different positions throughout the resin mass

(a) 1, 2, 3
(b) 2, 4, 5
(c) 1, 2, 5
(d) 1, 2, 4, 5
(e) all of the above

206. How is the marginal seal ensured when preparing a tooth for placement of a direct composite resin?

① place a topical fluoride solution on the margins of enamel and dentin
② etch the enamel and dentin margins of the preparation with manufacturer's solution of phosphoric acid, rinse and dry the tooth
③ use approximately 37 percent phosphoric acid solution for etching the enamel
④ use approximately 50 percent or more concentration of phosphoric acid to etch enamel margins

(a) 1, 3
(b) 2, 4
(c) 3, 4
(d) 1, 2, 3

207. If a patient's dental history includes high fluoride intake, the enamel etchant is left in place

(a) shorter than the average length of time
(b) longer than the average length of time
(c) the average length of time
(d) length of time does not matter

208. Which of the following apply to the placement of pit and fissure sealants on tooth surfaces

① tooth surfaces are cleaned with a fluoride polishing agent
② tooth surfaces are cleaned with a pumice wash abrasive
③ etchant is applied to enamel, left for 15 to 30 seconds, rinsed, and dried
④ light-curing white light is applied for 20 seconds to each tooth surface on which a sealant has been placed

(a) 1, 3
(b) 1, 4
(c) 2, 4
(d) 2, 3, 4

209. Which of the following actions should be taken if there are discrepancies in the depth of sealant coverage of the occlusal fossae and enamel margins?

① the tooth is re-etched for 30 seconds

② the tooth is re-etched for 60 seconds

③ the sealant is reapplied and cured for 60 seconds with a visible white light

④ the sealant is reduced using a round bur and a rubber polishing cup

    ⓐ 1, 3

    ⓑ 2, 3

    ⓒ 2, 4

    ⓓ 4 only

210. Where is the white curing light placed when curing the sealant material?

    ⓐ directly on the tooth surface

    ⓑ 1 mm from the tooth surface

    ⓒ 2 mm from the tooth surface

    ⓓ 5 mm from the tooth surface

211. Which of the following should be done if the enamel does NOT appear etched when rinsed and dried?

① polish the tooth enamel with slurry water

② expose the enamel to curing light

③ apply the sealant on dry enamel

④ reapply the phosphoric acid etchant

    ⓐ 1, 3

    ⓑ 2, 4

    ⓒ 1, 2, 3

    ⓓ 4 only

212. Which of the following correctly describe the method for applying tooth enamel sealant?

① a camel's hair brush is used

② material is placed on the occlusal surface only

③ a white curing light is used

④ eye shields are used by the operator and patient

    ⓐ 1, 3

    ⓑ 2, 4

    ⓒ 4 only

    ⓓ all of the above

213. Phosphoric acid etching liquid remains on the enamel for a minimum of
   (a) 15 seconds
   (b) 30 seconds
   (c) 45 seconds
   (d) 60 seconds

214. Angle Class II, division 1, differs from Angle Class II, division 2, in that
   (a) in division 1, the maxillary incisors are in linguoversion; in division 2, they are in labioversion
   (b) in division 1, the maxillary incisors are in labioversion; in division 2, the maxillary central incisors are in linguoversion
   (c) only in division 1 is there unilateral malocclusion
   (d) in division 2, the mandibular arch and body of the mandible are in a bilateral mesial relationship to the maxillary teeth

215. Rubbing etching solution on the enamel before direct bonding results in
   (a) fluorosis
   (b) quicker adherence of bonding material
   (c) removal of enamel tags
   (d) a caustic reaction

216. How soon after completion of final bonding of brackets may light force arch wire be placed?
   (a) 5 minutes
   (b) 15 minutes
   (c) 25 minutes
   (d) 40 minutes

217. Instruments used to place bonding material may be cleaned using
   (a) 70 percent alcohol
   (b) chloroform
   (c) hydrogen peroxide
   (d) oil of orange

218. Bonded brackets that have become loose may be replaced only after the
   (1) arch wires and ligature ties have been replaced
   (2) new bracket has been modified
   (3) enamel surface has been re-etched
   (4) tooth has been isolated with a rubber dam

Continued on next page

ⓐ 1, 2, 3
ⓑ 1, 3, 4
ⓒ 2, 3, 4
ⓓ 3, 4

219. Which of the following are true of elastic separators and their placement?

① dumbbell separators are applied to posterior teeth
② separators are placed to encircle the teeth at the contact areas
③ separators are seated with a seesaw motion
④ a separator must surround the contact on all sides
⑤ separators are placed when brackets are bonded

ⓐ 1, 2
ⓑ 1, 3, 4
ⓒ 2, 3, 4
ⓓ 2, 4, 5
ⓔ 3, 4, 5

220. Which of the following are true regarding the placement of TP spring separators?

① longer separators are used for molar contacts
② long beaked pliers are used for placement of all separators
③ the separator is inserted directly into the contact area
④ placement is from the lingual to the facial aspect

ⓐ 1, 2, 3
ⓑ 1, 2, 4
ⓒ 2, 3, 4
ⓓ 2, 4

221. Which of the following is true regarding the placement of brass wire separators?

ⓐ the appropriate wire size is 0.005
ⓑ placement is from facial to lingual
ⓒ the instrument of choice for placement is a hemostat
ⓓ after wire is wound, the free end is tucked occlusal to the contact area

222. Distal shoe-type appliances are

① removable
② fixed

③ used to maintain space

④ unilateral or bilateral

    ⓐ 1, 3

    ⓑ 1, 3, 4

    ⓒ 2, 3

    ⓓ 2, 3, 4

223. For each of the following numbered orthodontic procedures, select the appropriate category.

① correction of bad oral habits _____   ⓐ preventive

② space maintenance _____   ⓑ interceptive

③ serial extractions _____   ⓒ corrective

④ use of mechanical appliance _____

224. Identify the numbered cephalometric landmarks by matching their correct anatomic position with them.

① acanthion _____

② bregma _____

③ gnathion _____

④ zygion _____

⑤ pogonion _____

⑥ lambda _____

⑦ gonion _____

⑧ tragion _____

ⓐ the most lateral projection of the malar arch

ⓑ the lowest posterior point on an angle of the mandible

ⓒ the intersection of the sagittal and the lambdoidal sutures on the cranial vault

ⓓ the tip of the anterior nasal spine

ⓔ the lowest point of the median plane in the lower border of the chin

ⓕ the anterior prominence of the chin

ⓖ the anterior end of the sagittal suture

ⓗ the notch just above the tragus of the ear

225. Arch wires may be ligated with

① brass wire

② elastic rings

③ elastomeric chains

④ stainless steel wire

    ⓐ 1, 2

    ⓑ 1, 4

    ⓒ 2, 3

    ⓓ 2, 4

226. Instrumentation for a coronal polishing procedure includes

1. abrasive paste
2. right-angle handpiece
3. contra-angle handpiece
4. soft, flexible rubber cup
5. basic setup
6. dental floss or tape
7. mouth rinse

   a. 1, 3, 4, 6
   b. 1, 4, 6, 7
   c. 1, 2, 3, 4, 5, 6,
   d. all of the above

227. During coronal polishing, the revolving rubber cup is directed

1. from the free gingival groove
2. in overlapping strokes on the clinical crown
3. at the interproximal area
4. in overlapping strokes on the anatomic crown

   a. 1, 2
   b. 1, 3
   c. 1, 2, 3
   d. 1, 3, 4

228. As part of the coronal polishing procedure, the interproximal contact areas and embrasures are cleaned with

1. nonwaxed dental floss
2. fine-grit polishing strips
3. nonwaxed dental tape
4. a toothpick

   a. 1, 3
   b. 2, 4
   c. 1, 2, 3
   d. 3, 4

229. With the operator seated in the 9 o'clock position and the patient's head turned to the right during a coronal polishing procedure, which of the following tooth surfaces are accessible?

① facial of the maxillary left posterior quadrant

② lingual mandibular right posterior quadrant

③ facial of the mandibular left posterior quadrant

④ lingual of the maxillary right posterior quadrant

   ⓐ 1, 3

   ⓑ 2, 4

   ⓒ 3, 4

   ⓓ all of the above

230. To polish the lingual surfaces of the mandibular anteriors with a patient's head and chin tilted slightly upward, the

① patient's head is straight on the head rest

② right-angle handpiece is positioned from the side of the oral cavity

③ operator approaches the oral cavity from the 2 o'clock position

④ rubber cup on the handpiece is placed at the gingival margin of the lingual surface

   ⓐ 1, 2

   ⓑ 2, 4

   ⓒ 3, 4

   ⓓ 1, 2, 4

231. The pivotal area of the hand establishing and maintaining a fulcrum is the

   ⓐ little finger

   ⓑ fourth finger

   ⓒ index finger

   ⓓ thumb

232. During a coronal polishing procedure, the polishing cup is revolved slowly and

① directed to the gingiva from the occlusal surface

② directed to the gingiva from the incisal edge

③ moved constantly to prevent overheating of the enamel

④ with a stroking action, cup against the enamel

⑤ eased gently into the gingival sulcus

   ⓐ 1, 3

   ⓑ 2, 4

   ⓒ 3, 4, 5

   ⓓ 2, 3, 4, 5

233. The motion used to direct a right-angle handpiece and rubber cup with abrasive is

   ① stroking
   ② lifting
   ③ wiping
   ④ heavy

      ⓐ 1 only
      ⓑ 3 only
      ⓒ 1, 2, 3
      ⓓ 4 only

234. The abrasive for coronal polishing before placing acid etchant material on the tooth enamel must

      ⓐ be fluoride free
      ⓑ contain fluoride
      ⓒ be mixed with an oily base
      ⓓ be of a large particle size

235. Which of the following may be an effective treatment when the tooth crown is fractured and the dentinal third is involved?

   ① application of a palliative material to the crown
   ② application of intermediate restoration material
   ③ adaptation of a stainless steel crown
   ④ placement of a composite resin restoration

      ⓐ 1, 3
      ⓑ 2, 4
      ⓒ 1, 2, 3
      ⓓ 4 only

236. Which of the following are performed in a direct pulp capping procedure?

   ① calcium hydroxide powder placed on the pulp
   ② zinc oxide–eugenol placed over calcium hydroxide
   ③ a stainless steel crown placed over the crown
   ④ endodontic treatment to eradicate pulp

      ⓐ 1, 3
      ⓑ 2, 3
      ⓒ 1, 2, 3
      ⓓ 4 only

237. Which of the following appliances may be used to guide a tooth out of a locked position in the arch?

    ⓐ mouth guard

    ⓑ bite plane

    ⓒ splint

    ⓓ space maintainer

238. To fit correctly, a stainless steel crown must

    ① fit snugly on preparation and be 0.05 mm beneath the free gingival margin

    ② maintain facial-lingual, mesial-distal integrity in the dental arch

    ③ remain on plane with occlusal and marginal ridges of adjacent teeth

    ④ be stabilized with zinc phosphate cement

      ⓐ 1, 3

      ⓑ 2, 4

      ⓒ 1, 2, 3

      ⓓ 4 only

239. On recovery of the pulp of a traumatized tooth, which of the following treatments could be applied to rebuild the crown?

    ① stainless steel crown — zinc phosphate cement

    ② polycarbonate crown — calcium hydroxide plus zinc oxide – eugenol cement

    ③ acid-etched enamel — composite build-up

    ④ zinc phosphate cement — amalgam restoration

      ⓐ 1, 3

      ⓑ 2, 4

      ⓒ 1, 2, 3

      ⓓ 4 only

240. Which of the following materials are used for indirect pulp capping?

    ① calcium hydroxide

    ② zinc oxide – eugenol base

    ③ zinc phosphate cement

    ④ amalgam

      ⓐ 1, 3

      ⓑ 2, 4

      ⓒ 1, 2, 3

      ⓓ 2, 3, 4

241. Listed below are a series of steps necessary for effective sealant application. By use of the letters *a* through *g*, indicate the order of the procedure.

① isolate the tooth from salivary contamination ———

② apply an etching agent to the tooth surface ———

③ apply sealant material to the etched surface ———

④ explore the occlusal surface to check the integrity of the sealant ———

⑤ rinse the tooth surface with air-water spray for 10 seconds ———

⑥ carry out polishing of the surface to be sealed ———

⑦ evaluate the occlusion of the sealed surface ———

242. Listed below are a series of steps necessary for effective preventive resin restoration placement. By use of the letters *a* through *h*, indicate the order of the procedure.

① isolate the tooth from salivary contamination ———

② acid etch the occlusal surface ———

③ if necessary, apply additional sealant material ———

④ place a thin layer of resin bonding agent or dental bonding agent into the cavity preparation ———

⑤ place calcium hydroxide base on any exposed dentin ———

⑥ remove caries from isolated pits and fissures ———

⑦ carry out coronal polishing of the area to be treated ———

⑧ check the occlusion ———

243. When completing the setup for placement of a preventive resin restoration, the agent/tool of choice for removing isolated pits and fissures is

ⓐ a round bur in a high-speed handpiece

ⓑ a round bur in a low-speed handpiece

ⓒ a tapered diamond in a low-speed handpiece

ⓓ phosphoric acid applied with a fine brush

244. Ivory clamps, #8A or #14A, are used on a preschool patient to clamp

ⓐ cuspids

ⓑ premolars

ⓒ primary molars

ⓓ partially erupted permanent molars

ⓔ fully erupted permanent molars

245. A properly trimmed stainless steel crown should extend approximately how many millimeters below the gingival sulcus?

(a) 0.5

(b) 1.0

(c) 1.5 to 2.0

(d) 2.5

246. The instruments of choice for contouring the margins of a stainless steel crown
include

① #114 ball-and-socket pliers

② #137 Gordon pliers

③ #109 pliers

④ #k23 Ash pliers

(a) 1, 2

(b) 1, 3

(c) 2, 3

(d) 2, 4

247. The cervical margins of stainless steel crowns are crimped in order to

① achieve final close adaptation

② provide mechanical retention

③ protect the cement from oral fluids

④ maintain gingival health

⑤ restore the anatomic features of the natural crown

(a) 1, 2, 3

(b) 1, 3, 4

(c) 2, 3, 4

(d) 1, 2, 3, 4

(e) all of the above

248. Which of the following statements correctly describe the application of a rubber
dam on the right mandibular quadrant of a preschool patient?

① a 5 × 7-inch rubber dam is preferable

② a 5 × 5-inch rubber dam is preferable

③ the largest punch hole is used for the tooth to be clamped

④ holes are punched 1 mm apart

⑤ the primary first molar is the preferred tooth to be clamped

(a) 1, 3

(b) 2, 3

(c) 1, 2, 4

Continued on next page

ⓓ 2, 3, 4

ⓔ 3, 4, 5

249. Why are stannous fluoride and acidulated phosphate fluoride more effective than aqueous sodium fluoride?

① their pH is lower

② their mechanism of action is similar to ingested fluorides

③ they exhibit a greater fluoride reaction on the apatite crystal

④ they are much more stable

ⓐ 1, 2

ⓑ 1, 3

ⓒ 2, 3

ⓓ 3, 4

250. Which of the following statements is true in regard to the need for thorough coronal polishing before fluoride application?

ⓐ it is necessary because fluorides are less effective in the presence of dental plaque

ⓑ it is not necessary because the presence of plaque does not significantly reduce the agent's ability to penetrate it and deposit fluoride on the enamel

ⓒ it must be done to introduce a child to the sensation of the handpiece in the mouth

ⓓ decisions must be made on an individual basis

251. In addition to the basics, which of the following should be included in a tray setup for a formocreosol pulpotomy?

① cotton pellets

② fissure bur

③ #4, #6, or #8 round burs

④ excavator

⑤ paper points

⑥ Hedstrom file

ⓐ 1, 2, 3

ⓑ 1, 3, 4

ⓒ 1, 2, 3, 4

ⓓ 1, 2, 5, 6

ⓔ 2, 3, 5, 6

252. The solution of choice for removing debris from the root canal of primary teeth during the filing process is

    (a) sodium hypochlorite

    (b) 70 percent alcohol

    (c) distilled water

    (d) calcium chloride

253. To provide the strength and density needed in a finished denture, the acrylic resin and artificial teeth are placed in a rigid mold for curing

    (a) in a cold water bath

    (b) in a boiling water bath

    (c) on the laboratory bench

    (d) in a dry oven set at 305°F

254. Zinc phosphate cement is placed over calcium hydroxide

    (1) as an insulating base

    (2) in place of a temporary crown

    (3) as a luting agent

    (4) to contribute strength

    (5) to protect against thermal shock

        (a) 1, 2, 3

        (b) 1, 3, 4

        (c) 1, 4, 5

        (d) 2, 4, 5

255. To allow for the exothermic action of zinc phosphate cement on the glass slab, the mix is

    (a) spatulated deliberately in a figure-eight pattern

    (b) spatulated quickly and held in a mass on the slab

    (c) accomplished in 3 minutes

    (d) accomplished in 30 seconds

256. Zinc phosphate cement mixed for an insulating base should be of what viscosity?

    (a) thin

    (b) watery

    (c) medium

    (d) puttylike

257. After cementation of a permanent cast crown, the excess cement is removed

  ① by using an explorer

  ② by flushing the tooth with copious amounts of water

  ③ before final set of cement

  ④ after evaluation of the occlusion

     ⓐ 1 only

     ⓑ 1, 3

     ⓒ 2, 4

     ⓓ 4 only

258. Recommended manipulation of zinc oxide–eugenol cement for temporary coverage would include which of the following?

  ① mixing to medium viscosity

  ② mixing using a small flexible spatula and paper pad

  ③ cleaning the tooth preparation with isopropyl alcohol before cementation

  ④ incorporating zinc acetate crystals to accelerate the set

  ⑤ setting in 5 to 7 minutes

     ⓐ 1, 3

     ⓑ 2, 3

     ⓒ 1, 2, 4

     ⓓ 1, 2, 5

259. Use letters in alphabetic order to indicate the correct sequence for use of a transistorized pulp vitalometer, leaving blank those steps that do not apply

  ① isolate the tooth to be tested with cotton rolls and dry ＿＿＿

  ② begin the test with the rheostat set at 0 ＿＿＿

  ③ apply prophy paste to the facial or lingual isolated tooth ＿＿＿

  ④ place the conductive tip on the middle of the facial or lingual surface ＿＿＿

  ⑤ increase the current rapidly if the conductive tip is placed on filling material ＿＿＿

260. Which of the following instruments is NOT placed on a routine endodontic tray for a cleaning and shaping procedure?

     ⓐ endodontic explorer

     ⓑ 5- to 6-ml Luer-Lok syringe

     ⓒ Glick #1

     ⓓ barbed broach

261. Which of the following is true of chelators?

    ⓐ they work quickly

    ⓑ they remove canal obstructions to allow passage of instruments

    ⓒ they should be placed in the canals only after instrumentation has occurred

    ⓓ in order to soften dentin, they should remain in canals for several hours

262. Percussion is performed on a tooth to ascertain

    ⓐ the mobility of a tooth

    ⓑ a tooth's sensitivity

    ⓒ whether or not a fracture is complete

    ⓓ whether or not there is a variation in translucency between teeth

263. Identify the instruments shown in the figure below by placing the correct letter after the name

    ① curved gutta percha plugger _____   ⑤ file _____

    ② smooth broach _____   ⑥ rat-tail file _____

    ③ reamer _____   ⑦ barbed broach _____

    ④ straight gutta percha plugger _____   ⑧ Hedstrum file _____

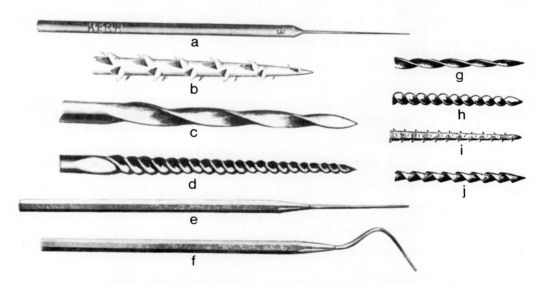

(From Torres H, Ehrlich A: Modern Dental Assisting, 4th ed. Philadelphia, WB Saunders, 1990, p 669)

264. A three-way syringe may be used to

① spray water

② blow air

③ deliver a combination of air and water

④ retract tissue

    ⓐ 1, 2, 3

    ⓑ 1, 3, 4

    ⓒ 2, 3, 4

    ⓓ all of the above

265. Preformed orthodontic bands are characterized by their

① shapes designed to fit specific teeth

② specific designs for mandibular and maxillary teeth

③ bibeveled gingival edges

④ cleats on the distolingual surface

    ⓐ 1, 2

    ⓑ 1, 3

    ⓒ 1, 2, 4

    ⓓ 3, 4

266. The distance from the incisal edge of a banded maxillary central to the bracket slot should be approximately

    ⓐ 2.5 mm

    ⓑ 3.5 mm

    ⓒ 4.5 mm

    ⓓ 5.0 mm

267. The instrument generally used for the initial seating of a band on a tooth is

    ⓐ How pliers

    ⓑ a Schure instrument

    ⓒ a mallet and chisel

    ⓓ a band seater

268. An asymmetric open bite is secondary to what habit?

    ⓐ thumb sucking

    ⓑ tongue thrusting

    ⓒ tongue sucking

    ⓓ mouth breathing

269. How is a preformed arch wire placed?

  (a) first place one end into the tube slot on a banded right molar
  (b) first place one end into the tube slot on the banded left molar
  (c) both ends are seated into the tube slots simultaneously
  (d) both ends are first placed in the right and left premolar brackets

270. How is a custom wedge placed when securing a circumferential matrix band?

  (1) on the gingival floor at the proximal surface
  (2) always from the facial surface
  (3) at the gingival embrasure
  (4) at the height of the contour of the matrix band

   (a) 1, 3
   (b) 2, 4
   (c) 1, 2, 3
   (d) 4 only

271. Which of the following materials are suitable for custom wedges used to secure matrix bands?

  (1) wood
  (2) acrylic
  (3) plastic
  (4) metal

   (a) 1, 3
   (b) 2, 4
   (c) 1, 2, 3
   (d) 4 only

272. A matrix band for a Class II three-surface amalgam restoration must encompass the tooth tightly at the gingiva to

  (1) provide sufficient bulk of material for carving
  (2) make carving more accessible
  (3) provide sufficient contours for the contact areas
  (4) prevent excessive amalgam from being pushed beyond the gingival margin

   (a) 1, 2
   (b) 1, 3
   (c) 1, 3, 4
   (d) 2, 3, 4

273. When removing an arch wire, a Schure instrument is used to

    (a) free the pigtail from the bracket

    (b) hold the ligature wire

    (c) cut the ligature wire

    (d) pull the arch wire free of the brackets

274. For which schedule of drugs do dentists NOT have to include the controlled substances permit number?

    (a) schedule I

    (b) schedule II

    (c) schedule III

    (d) schedule IV

    (e) schedule V

275. Which one of the following is an anxiolytic agent?

    (a) Demerol

    (b) morphine

    (c) aspirin

    (d) Valium

276. Type II gypsum material is referred to as

    (1) plaster of Paris

    (2) dental stone

    (3) laboratory plaster

    (4) die stone

        (a) 1, 3

        (b) 2, 4

        (c) 1, 2, 3

        (d) 4 only

277. Cavity varnishes placed in a cavity preparation cannot be expected to

    (a) minimize marginal leakage

    (b) act as thermal insulators

    (c) prevent acids from zinc phosphate cements from penetrating the pulp

    (d) prevent corrosion from amalgam restorations from penetrating the pulp

Questions 278 through 280 refer to the chart below.

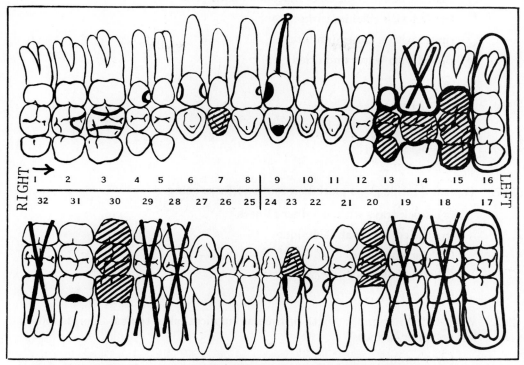

(From Torres H, Ehrlich A: Modern Dental Assisting, 4th ed. Philadelphia, WB Saunders, 1990, p 467)

278. Which of the following describes the symbol placed on the root of tooth # 9?

(a) root canal prepared for filling

(b) endodontic treatment pending

(c) root canal filled

(d) dowel pin placed

279. Teeth numbered 14, 18, 19, 28, 29, and 32 are

(a) missing

(b) marked for extraction

(c) a bridge abutment

(d) a bridge pontic

280. Teeth numbered 15 and 30 are restored with

(a) full gold crowns

(b) full porcelain crowns

(c) amalgam restorations

(d) temporary steel crowns

281. Before the application of topical fluoride gel, the teeth are
    ① cleaned with a fluoride or silicone dioxide paste
    ② treated with calcium carbonate
    ③ rinsed with a caries inhibitor
    ④ rinsed with water and dried
        ⓐ 1, 2
        ⓑ 1, 4
        ⓒ 2, 3
        ⓓ 2, 4

282. Topical fluoride gel is placed on tooth surfaces using
    ⓐ stock trays with absorbent liners
    ⓑ the cotton swab technique
    ⓒ a spray bottle
    ⓓ a rubber polishing cup

283. What is the minimum length of time an application of topical fluoride must be left on tooth surfaces?
    ⓐ 1 minute
    ⓑ 2 minutes
    ⓒ 3 minutes
    ⓓ 4 minutes

284. After the application of topical fluoride, patients are cautioned
    ⓐ not to swallow the excess material
    ⓑ not to drink or eat for a minimum of 30 minutes
    ⓒ to rinse their mouth with saline solution
    ⓓ to return to the office if the material sloughs off

285. Removable prostheses are polished by the use of
    ① abrasive pumice
    ② a bristle brush
    ③ a fresh rag wheel
    ④ tripoli on a rag wheel
        ⓐ 1, 2
        ⓑ 2, 3
        ⓒ 3, 4
        ⓓ 4 only

286. What is used to clean a removable partial denture?

① hand instruments
② a solution of sodium hypochlorite
③ sandpaper disks
④ an ultrasonic cleaner

ⓐ 1 only
ⓑ 2 only
ⓒ 1, 3
ⓓ 2, 4

287. Which of the following steps is necessary before placing a periodontal dressing in the presence of sutures?

ⓐ check the sutures for tension
ⓑ snip sutures but leave in place
ⓒ apply alcohol to the area
ⓓ apply petroleum jelly to the sutures

288. What are the responsibilities of the dentist and staff members when a patient under treatment dies in the dental office?

① notify the next of kin
② call paramedics
③ alter the patient's original records to prove that the patient was instructed to see a physician before treatment
④ notify the coroner's office
⑤ notify the state board of dentistry

ⓐ 1, 2, 3
ⓑ 1, 3, 5
ⓒ 1, 2, 4, 5
ⓓ all of the above

289. Which of the following steps should be taken to construct a custom temporary crown?

① obtain a "snap" alginate impression before the tooth is prepared
② lubricate the tooth to be prepared and cover the crown with self-polymerizing acrylic
③ place an alginate impression containing acrylic on the tooth prepared for a crown
④ contour acrylic to the shape of the tooth and allow to cure
⑤ remove the crown from the impression, trim excess acrylic "flash," check the crown for fit on the prepared tooth

Continued on next page

(a) 1, 2
(b) 1, 3
(c) 2, 4
(d) 1, 3, 5

290. Which of the following applies to the removal of continuous sutures?

① cut the suture 2 mm beyond the knot
② grasp the knot with pliers and pull the suture through the tissue
③ grasp the length of the cut suture and pull through the tissue
④ grasp the vertical suture loops and remove them from the tissue

(a) 1, 3
(b) 1, 4
(c) 2, 4
(d) 1, 2, 3

Rationale for
Test Questions
TEST II

Rationale for Test Questions
TEST II

ANSWERS AND RATIONALE:

1. ⓓ When gathering information and data for *new* patients, before treatment, patients should be asked about regular medications (prescribed and over-the-counter drugs) taken, any congenital and chronic conditions, the amount and frequency of exposure to ionizing radiation, and any history of adverse reactions to local or general anesthesia. *Repeat* patients should be questioned about any changes in health and about reactions to medications since last visiting the dental practice.

2. ⓑ To hear and obtain a patient's blood pressure using a stethoscope, the disk of the stethoscope must be placed at the antecubital fossa just above the bend at the inner side of the elbow (it is placed on the brachial artery in this position).

3. ⓑ To obtain an accurate temperature reading, a thermometer must be read immediately after removal from a patient's mouth; otherwise, the thermometer may change.

4. ⓒ Herpes simplex virus type 1 (HSV-1), aphthous ulcer (canker sore), and herpes simplex virus type 2 (HSV-2) are contagious. Any abnormal tissues observed must be called to the attention of the dentist.

5. ⓒ Ankylosis is a condition in which the alveolar bone attaches itself directly to the cementum of the tooth. The periodontium is absent.

6. ⓐ Decreased salivary function caused by disease, possibly medications, or radiation therapy adversely affects the gingiva and other tissues, thus exposing the roots of the teeth to the development and progression of root caries.

7. ⓒ The schedules of pharmaceuticals controlled by the Food and Drug Administration (FDA) are designated as controlled substances I through V. Substances in these classifications are eligible for review by federal agents if a complaint is filed with the FDA.

8. ⓒ Schedule II drugs including codeine, opium, oxycodone (Percodan), morphine, and barbiturates have medical/dental usefulness. An inventory of these drugs is subject to review.

9. ⓑ In the private practice of dentistry, dentists are permitted to personally dispense controlled substances to their patients. A dental assistant may dispense drugs to patients under the direct supervision of a dentist. A record is kept of the drugs dispensed, along with an inventory (purchased and dispensed) of each medication.

162

10. (a) The objective in mixing the base and catalyst of the elastomer impression materials is to obtain homogeneity and a uniform cure of the mix.

11. (c) Obtaining an acceptable impression using elastomeric impression material in a custom tray depends on use of peripheral wax on the margin of the tray and tray adhesive on the inner surfaces.

12. (c) Zinc oxide–eugenol cement used as an insulating base is placed over a liner of calcium hydroxide to protect the pulp.

13. (a) Copal varnish (two coats) is placed carefully in the cavity preparation immediately before placement of the metallic restoration. The varnish forms a seal and reduces the possibility of microleakage between margins of the enamel and the metallic restoration.

14. (c) To insulate the pulp from thermal shock under conductive-type restorative material (e.g., amalgam, gold), zinc oxide–eugenol, light-cured glass ionomers, and carboxylates are used.

15. (c) Calcium hydroxide insulates the pulp of a traumatized tooth and encourages the pulp to lay down new odontoblasts, forming a new layer of dentin.

16. (b) The sequence of use of dental materials to restore a tooth with a traumatized pulp is as follows: calcium hydroxide, cavity varnish, zinc oxide–eugenol, polycarboxylate cement, and silver amalgam.

17. (b) To lute (cement) orthodontic appliances directly to tooth enamel, an orthodontist may use silicophosphate and polycarboxylate cements. Note: The enamel is first slightly etched to receive the bracket, which is cemented directly to the etched surface.

18. (d) Generic formulas of glass ionomer are adapted to dentistry in the form of luting agents, cavity liners, Class I and II restorations, core build-up for cast restorations, and light-cured restorative systems.

19. (d) Because ethoxybenzoic acid (EBA) cement reduces microleakage at the margins of a cast restoration and tooth enamel, it may be used for permanent cementation.

20. (d) Polycarboxylate (polyacrylate) cement, referred to as *carboxylate cement*, contains modified zinc oxide and magnesium oxide and may be placed under amalgam or composite restorations.

21. (b) Visible light–activated elastomer impression material is a single-component system and is purchased as light or heavy bodied. The light-bodied material is usually used for syringe adaptation around the tooth preparation, and the heavy-bodied mix is placed in the impression tray.

22. (c) Glass ionomer cement may be used to cement cast posts and cores, orthodontic bands, and cast crowns.

23. (b) Glass ionomer cement is used for post and core and build-up in crown and bridge restorations.

24. (c) To prepare a prepackaged capsule of glass ionomer cement, the knob is twisted from the end of the capsule, the opened capsule is placed in a hand-held applicator, and the cement mix is squeezed into the tooth preparation.

25. (c) Insulating base of calcium hydroxide is placed level with the surface of the axial wall, level with the pulpal floor, and covering any indentations of the preparation near the pulpal area.

26. (a) Slabs and spatulas for mixing cements must be dry and at 68°F, particularly the glass slab and spatula for zinc phosphate cement.

27. (c) Cavity varnishes of one or more resins may be placed in a deep cavity preparation before the insulating base, as well as over bases containing calcium hydroxide or zinc oxide–eugenol. All of these materials are palliative to the tooth structures.

28. (a) Dentin is conditioned with 10 percent polyacrylic acid to achieve maximum bonding before placing glass ionomer restorative material.

29. (d) Braided retraction cord is the material of choice to be placed to retract the gingival tissue around the finish line of a tooth prepared for a cast restoration. The braided cord is removed immediately before the impression is taken.

30. (a) To obtain a bite registration, vinyl polysiloxane impression material or wax with metallic filings is used.

31. (c) Deterioration of a packaged drug commonly is identified by its change of color.

32. (e) Drug-dependent individuals usually have a poor diet; some consume excessive amounts of refined carbohydrates; some have a dry mouth; and some bruxate. All of these factors contribute to various dental problems.

33. (a) Cephalosporins, erythromycin, and ampicillin are antibiotics that are chemically related to penicillins. Nystatin is an antifungal agent.

34. (c) When ordering narcotics for the office supply, two copies of each order must be sent to the supplier and a third must be filed in the office's narcotics record.

35. (d) Condensers that may be used to pack gutta percha points into prepared canals are the lateral, vertical, and end condensers and the universal Wesco condenser.

36. (b) The sequence in operating a transistorized pulp vitalometer is to isolate and dry the tooth to be tested, apply prophy paste to the facial or lingual

surface of the suspect tooth, and begin the test with contact on the enamel and the rheostat set at zero.

37. ⓓ A lentulo spatula is a twisted wire instrument used in the slow-speed handpiece to spin filling materials into root canals.

38. ⓒ Gates-Glidden burs are available in six sizes, and each bur is marked at its latch attachment portion with an indented stripe to indicate the size.

39. ⓑ In the situation described in the question, an accurate radiograph is necessary.

40. ⓑ Files #8 and #10 should not be placed in the canal when exposing working length radiographs because the small tips may not show on a radidograph.

41. ⓐ Broaches are made with tiny barbs pulled from the instrument shaft and are not used for enlarging and shaping.

42. ⓒ Both a Gates-Glidden file and a Peeso reamer have noncutting tips, but a Peeso reamer has parallel sides whereas a Gates-Glidden has an elliptic shape.

43. ⓓ An endodontic explorer may be used to stimulate carious dentin directly to test responsiveness, as well as to locate canal orifices.

44. ⓐ Pluggers are flat at the working end, whereas spreaders are pointed.

45. ⓓ Obturating materials extending beyond the apex are irritants and affect healing.

46. ⓓ If a root canal master cone appears buckled on a radiograph, it is too small. A larger cone should be selected.

47. ⓐ Apicoectomy is necessary if filling material extrudes out of the apex and a root canal procedure fails to heal.

48. ⓒ Retrofilling is a method of filling the root canal from the apical area of the tooth using a Messing root canal gun.

49. ⓓ Zinc-free silver alloy is used in retrofilling because it does not react with any moisture present in the root canal.

50. ⓒ Needles used for administration can be contaminated with human immunodeficiency virus.

51. ⓔ ⓑ ⓕ ⓖ ⓐ ⓗ

52. ⓑ ⓒ ⓐ ⓓ

53. ⓓ Routine infection control should assume that all patients are high risk.

54. (b) The Occupational Safety and Health Administration (OSHA) requirements specify that confidential medical records be kept for all employees at risk of blood-borne pathogen transmission in the dental office setting; all dental patients should be treated as though they are HIV and hepatitis B virus (HBV) infected; and employers provide HBV vaccine at no charge to employees who are at risk of HBV infection.

55. (a) All instruments must be examined for the presence of bioburden after removal from the ultrasonic cleaner.

56. (d) The common characteristic that surface disinfectants such as diluted iodophors, synthetic phenols, and chlorines have is that they are effective surface cleaners.

57. (c) Regarding employees who may come in contact with blood, OSHA states that employers are responsible for preparing a written exposure central plan; providing free hepatitis vaccinations; providing barriers such as gloves, masks, shields, and smocks; and identifying workers who may be at risk.

58. (d) According to OSHA guidelines, tasks performed by dental office employees are categorized as I, II, and III.

59. (a) Foil is not used as a protective barrier for the head of an x-ray machine because of its tendency to tear.

60. (b) (d) (a) (c)

61. (b) Three common problems related to diminished efficiency of office sterilization procedures are operator error, improper preparation or wrapping of instruments, and defective control gauges on the steam autoclave or dry heat sterilizer.

62. (d) Holding solutions for soiled instruments begin microbial kill, prevent airborne transmission of dried microorganisms, minimize handling of soiled instruments, and prevent blood, saliva, and debris from drying on soiled instruments.

63. (c) When only outer surfaces of handpieces are cleaned and exposed to disinfectants, the inner portion of the handpiece is *not* disinfected. It is advised that the handpiece be taken apart and sterilized in a steam autoclave.

64. (e) Disposable face masks make it more difficult to transmit oral pathogens, a 95 percent filtration of small particles. A face mask and shield fully prevent the transmission of respiratory pathogens. Face masks are also recommended to cover the nasal mucosa.

65. 1: (b) (c) ; 2: (a) (b) (c) (d) (e) ; 3: (a) (b) (c) (d) (e) ; 4: (c) ;

   5: (a) (b) (c) ; 6: (b) (c) (e) ; 7: (b) (c) (e)

66. ⓓ Protocol for infection control for partial or complete dentures in the dental laboratory includes the following: disinfect new prostheses before packaging; discard, launder, or autoclave used polishing rag wheels after each use; use fresh pumice for each polishing procedure; place finished/polished prostheses in moist, sealed bags.

67. ⓑ ⓙ ⓔ ⓖ ⓘ ⓗ ⓓ

68. ⓑ Capping a used needle prevents a needle-stick injury. Placing the guard on the tray and placing the needle into the guard contributes to the prevention of needle-stick injury.

69. ⓓ A 1-inch needle is used for infiltration anesthesia, and a 1 5/8-inch needle is used for block anesthesia. *Gauge* refers to the thickness of the needle, with the thickness diminishing as the numbers become higher.

70. ⓓ To be effective, local anesthetic solution must be deposited into the intraosseous area near the tooth. This technique is advantageous in that it provides anesthesia to tissues where other types of anesthesia do not. It is used to provide anesthesia for an individual tooth.

71. ⓑ Neo-Cobefrin has an astringent effect to retain the anesthetic solution in an area without overstimulating the heart.

72. ⓒ One procedure used when handling a syringe in a safe manner includes recapping the needle after check of solution, placing the ring of the syringe on the operator's thumb, and turning the lumen (bevel of the needle) toward the alveolus.

73. ⓒ A firm tap of the ring or base of the syringe is necessary to attach the harpoon to the rubber plunger; harpoon attachment is checked by retracting the plunger; droplets of anesthetic solution are expelled to ensure that the needle is not obstructed; then the needle cover should be cautiously replaced to prevent needle-stick injury.

74. ⓓ To obtain anesthesia of the dental tissues on a side of the face and oral cavity, the anesthetic solution is deposited near the plexus of the trigeminal nerve. Note: the trigeminal nerve provides innervation to the right or left side of the oral cavity and face.

75. ⓒ A vasoconstrictor decreases blood flow; thus, it delays systemic absorption of the anesthetic solution into the system. It also prolongs the effect of the anesthetic and decreases bleeding in the injected area during surgical procedures.

76. ⓐ Topical anesthetic ointment is placed on dried oral mucosa at the planned site of an injection before injecting the solution because it temporarily numbs the nerve endings in the mucosa and remains effective approximately 3 to 5 minutes.

77. ⓓ Every precaution must be taken for the protection of the patient and the operating team when adminstering general anesthesia.

78. ⓒ Contamination of the anesthetic solution is often due to the alcohol used to sterilize the anesthetic Carpules. Paresthesia may be total or partial, and it usually resolves in about 8 weeks without treatment. Trauma of the nerve sheath is usually of mechanical origin. Hemorrhage in the area of the nerve sheath could be due to a prolonged surgical procedure.

79. ⓐ The planes of analgesia (Plane I and Plane II) are safe for dental procedures because patients can remain alert and responsive to a dentist's directions and recover quickly from the effect of analgesia when the dental procedure is concluded.

80. ⓒ At baseline, a patient remains conscious and cooperative but is very relaxed, with protective reflexes intact and active. Vital signs remain normal.

81. ⓐ To anesthetize the maxillary central incisors, topical anesthetic ointment is swabbed on the facial mucosa opposite the apices of the teeth. After 3 minutes, using a short needle and a syringe, local anesthetic solution is deposited in the facial mucosa into the alveolus in alignment with the apices of the maxillary central incisors. The anterior branch of the superior alveolar nerve is affected by this injection. In some instances, an anterior palatal injection is made into the area supplied by the incisive nerve.

82. ⓐ A block injection is used to effect anesthesia of a mandibular first molar, so a 1 5/8-inch-long 27-gauge needle is used.

83. ⓒ The right second premolar is tooth #29; therefore, depositing anesthetic solution near the left mandibular foramen would be incorrect — the wrong side of the oral cavity.

84. ⓐ Local anesthetic agents in use today are amides developed since the synthesis of lidocaine (Xylocaine), and they are relatively free of allergic effects. The current group of local anesthetic agents includes mepivacaine (Carbocaine), priolocaine (Citanest), bupivacaine (Marcaine), and etidocaine (Duranest). Local anesthetic agents are described in terms of their potency, the concentration required to produce the required effect of anesthesia, their onset time, the time necessary to penetrate the nerve fiber and cause conduction block, and their duration of effect to cover the working time for a given procedure. For example, mepivacaine, 2 percent concentration, giving intermediate potency, provides 50 to 140 minutes duration of anesthesia in the tissues.

85. ⓒ Normally, the onset of a local anesthetic is within 10 to 20 seconds.

86. ⓒ A carrier may have been exposed to a disease but not yet have the obvious symptoms, may have recovered from the disease, or may have been exposed to the disease but not become ill, and may still harbor specific organisms and be capable of transmitting the disease to others. A carrier always remains a carrier, and because this condition may be difficult to detect, all patients should be treated as carriers.

87. ⓒ Diabetic acidosis may lead to a coma, convulsions, or death.

88. (a) An initial purpose of inflammation is to destroy the causative agent and to remove it and its by-products from the body. If it is not successful in this, it may limit the extension of the causative agent and its harmful effects throughout the body.

89. (e) Using finger pressure placed at the side of the sternocleidomastoid muscle or the recessed area near the clavicle, the carotid pulse is detected.

90. (d) A finger sweep is performed on an unconscious patient before cardiopulmonary resuscitation (CPR) to attempt removal of a lodged object and is followed by an abdominal thrust to ensure dislodgment of the object, providing a clear field for resuscitation.

91. (b) The advantages of two-rescuer CPR are that 100 compressions per minute can be attained, thus providing more blood and oxygen flow to the brain. A patient's lungs are more quickly ventilated by the delivery of two breaths per compression.

92. (b) Anaphylactic shock is a sudden reaction to an allergen; it can be life threatening. The condition may occur immediately as the cells release histamines. The capillaries are dilated, and plasma and other fluids entering the body tissues cause edema and thus lowered vascular output. Also, a rash and itching frequently occur together with large welts.

93. (d) A patient who has been in a supine or subsupine position (head lower than knees) for a long time experiences hypoxemia in the brain if suddenly raised to an upright position. To equalize the flow of blood to the extremities and the brain, slowly positioning the patient upright is recommended. This condition occurs more frequently in elderly patients.

94. (b) If a foreign object is visible in the oropharynx, an attempt is made to dislodge it with a finger sweep; if the patient is coughing and can speak, the finger sweep is not indicated. With the patient standing, the abdominal thrust could be performed to dislodge the foreign object.

95. (b) Substernal pain is a result of narrowing of the coronary arteries and decreased blood to the heart. Radiating pain may be located in the arms and chest. Cyanosis is common in angina attacks. Patients may have temporary swelling of the ankles and hands and shortness of breath. They may feel anxious and express a desire to be seated in an upright position.

96. (d) A patient suffering an attack of angina pectoris is seated in an upright position, administered one nitroglycerin tablet (Note: Patients with a tendency to have angina pectoris usually carry prescribed nitroglycerin) placed under the tongue, and administered 100 percent oxygen until the paramedics arrive and he or she is more comfortable.

97. (d) A patient suffering pulmonary arrest has ceased breathing, and emergency artificial respiration must be immediately initiated. The basic procedure for artificial ventilation should be followed.

98. (c) Diabetic acidosis is a condition brought on by a patient's disregard of fixed medication and food intake schedules. A diabetic patient's general health condition may be considered "brittle" by his or her physician; therefore, all directions must be followed.

99. (a) Patients suffering symptoms of insulin shock (hypoglycemia) may have received their prescribed dose of insulin but not have eaten. First aid may include placing a sugar cube under the tongue or giving a conscious patient a glass of orange juice. Patients are constantly monitored until fully recovered from this condition. A physician may be called if response to this treatment is not immediate.

100. (c) A Class III injury is an extensive fracture of the crown exposing the pulp of the tooth. It may be treated by placing calcium hydroxide, zinc oxide–eugenol, or intermediary restorative material over the tooth within a temporary crown form.

101. (c) Before providing first aid measures for an unconscious person, a rescuer assesses whether the patient has an open airway, if he or she is breathing, and whether a pulse can be felt. If these vital signs are absent, the rescuer calls for help and, beginning with a finger sweep, positions the patient for abdominal thrust or CPR.

102. (c) To obtain an accurate impression of a tooth preparation for a cast restoration, retraction cord is placed within the gingival sulcus. Using elastomeric impression materials, the retraction cord is removed (counterclockwise from its placement) immediately before the impression material is extruded from the syringe.

103. (a) There are three different types of resin polymerization: (1) autopolymerizing, which takes place when the monomer and polymer are mixed together; (2) heat cured, in which heat under pressure is required for polymerization; and (3) light cured, in which resins polymerize when exposed to either visible or ultraviolet light for a proper length of time. The advantages of light-cured resins are that no mixing is required; thus, there is no exposure to monomer fumes and curing heat is not needed. Their working time is unlimited, and they cure to a smooth, hard surface.

104. (c) Materials placed within an ill-fitting denture must provide a cushioning effect to the traumatized tissues of the dental arch. All of the temporary spongy-type resins, reliners, or conditioners meet these criteria.

105. (d) To provide an even and adequate space for impression material when fabricating a custom tray, at least two layers of base plate wax are placed over the cast before placing the malleable custom tray material.

106. (c) Adhesion of the material to an impression tray is imperative when the material is removed from the mouth. An impression detached from the tray would be distorted. Because perforated trays used for amalgamation are not practical as custom-built trays, adhesion can best be obtained by applying an adhesive to a solid tray. Adhesive cements provided with the various types of rubber impression materials differ and are *not* interchangeable.

107. (b) A container of dental supplies received is usually accompanied by an itemized list of the supplies shipped and their cost. This item is referred to as an *invoice*. If the supplies are received with a list only, this is referred to as a *packing slip*.

108. (c) To officially complete payment, the payee (the person to whom the check is written) must endorse the check before receiving cash or passing it on as payment.

109. (b) Until a bank clears the amount of deposits in transit to the account, the amount is added to the bank statement.

110. (c) In the problem described in the question, 20 percent of $750 is $150, and 8 percent of $750 is $60. Sixty dollars plus $150 is $210, which is subtracted from $750.

111. (b) The employer's contribution matches the employee's.

112. (d) The percentage of withholding tax is determined by a scale obtained from the federal government. The amount withheld must be forwarded to the Internal Revenue Service (IRS) district office each quarter.

113. (d) The Uniform Code in Dental Procedures and Nomenclature was developed by the American Dental Association (ADA) to speed and simplify the reporting of dental procedures on claims.

114. (b) When amalgam alloys containing zinc are contaminated by water, hydrogen is produced by electrolytic action. The hydrogen collects within the restoration and increases the internal pressure to levels high enough to cause the amalgam to creep and produce expansion.

115. (d) A custom matrix band must be secured and firmly held in place to withstand the placement, condensing, and carving of amalgam. To effectively secure the custom matrix, a custom wedge is preferred.

116. (c) The wedge and matrix are carefully removed from a freshly placed amalgam to avoid fracturing the mass. The wedge is removed lingually, and the matrix is carefully moved away from the restoration and lifted upward.

117. (b) A Class V cavity is located at the gingival third of the facial surface and would not require a matrix band or an interproximal instrument. A cervical clamp could be used for gingival tissue displacement.

118. (a) When placing a Tofflemire matrix and wedge, the retainer is placed parallel to the facial surfaces of the teeth, the matrix band extends approximately 1 mm above the occlusal margin of the prepared tooth, and the gingival area of the band extends approximately 0.5 to 1.0 mm beyond the margin of the preparation.

119. (b) Implants engage cortical bone because it is more dense and stable and it allows cancellous-type bone to fill in the spaces around and into the perforations of the metallic implant. Cortical bone is compact, hard, and strong and provides a suitable base to withstand the stresses placed on implants.

120. (c) Hypertension per se should not be a contraindication to implants. Absolute or relative contraindications to implant therapy include uncontrolled endocrine conditions such as diabetes, a high risk for endocarditis, such as in patients with artificial heart valves, psychiatric disorders, osteoporosis, connective tissue disorders, immunosuppression, chronic steroid therapy, chronic alcoholism, and cigarette smoking, as well as persons for whom a lower success rate may be expected. A lack of commitment to oral hygiene and follow-up care also contributes to a poor success rate, because optimal healing and tissue regeneration are not possible under these conditions.

121. 1: (b) ; 2: (d) ; 3: (a) . *Endo* means "within" or "inward"; *trans* means "through," "across," or "beyond"; and *sub* means "below" or "under."

122. (d) A periodontist is responsible for treating peri-implantitis because of the many similarities in the management of periodontitis and peri-implantitis.

123. (b) Chlorhexidine rinses work effectively to control peri-implant plaque accumulation with associated peri-implant gingivitis. Because chlorhexidine can be associated with calculus build-up, its routine application should not be required if home care is effective without it.

124. (c) The use of sonic or ultrasonic instruments to scale around implants is not recommended because they may cause scratches and irregularities on the implant surfaces, potentiate plaque accumulation, and lead to inflammation. Teflon, plastic, wooden, or possibly gold tipped instruments are recommended for scaling. Some manufacturers place markers on plastic instruments to indicate the number of times they may be autoclaved.

125. (d) Patients are advised against using hard brushes or any metals to clean implants. End-tufted brushes, floss, yarn, interdental brushes with nylon-coated wires, water picks, or other oral irrigators are recommended.

126. (d) Depending on the molar to be prepared, an assistant places the aspirating tip out of the operator's line of vision. It may be placed at the facial surface of the left mandibular molar, thus retracting the cheek. The opening of the vacuum tip is placed along the facial surface of the tooth. Alternatively, the aspirating tip may be placed at the lingual area across the tongue, depressing the tongue.

127. (a) The post occupies one-third of the diameter of the root canal. It is the same length as the overall length of the tooth crown. The size of the post should resist tipping forces on the crown, which could cause it to bend or fracture.

128. (b) In fixed bridgework, keyway slots in the preparation of a dowel post and core indicate the path of insertion and prevent the dowel from loosening and from turning or tipping when cemented in the prepared canal space. These slots are made in the dentin next to the canal.

129. (b) A paste bite registration is performed in the sequence listed in answer *b* in the question.

130. (b) To maintain integrity of the arch and to protect the prepared teeth, temporary crowns (temporary coverage) on posterior prepared teeth must contact adjacent teeth and maintain occlusal function. A tight margin aids in mechanical retention of the crown, protection of the cement from oral fluids, and maintenance of good gingival health.

131. (c) Moistened Styrofoam sheets (10 to 25 mm) or strips are used to create space for impression material when constructing a custom tray. The width of the Styrofoam layer is adjusted to provide the necessary thickness for the impression material.

132. (f) (b) (c) (a) (d) (e)

The framework is the metal skeleton, usually constructed of gold alloy or chromium, that provides basic support for the saddle with the connectors; the bar serves as a connector; the stress breaker serves to relieve the abutment teeth from excessive occlusal loads and stresses; the saddle rests on the oral mucosa covering the alveolar ridge and retains the acrylic teeth; the metal clasps help support and provide stability to the partial denture; the rest is the metal projection on or near the clasp of the partial and is designed to control the extent of the seating of the partial and prevent its moving gingivally.

133. (c) Bite registrations are essential to indicate the relationship of teeth in the arch to the prepared tooth *and* the vertical relationship and dimension with opposing teeth.

134. (c) An overdenture has recessed areas that snap over copings that have been cemented into endodontically treated teeth.

135. (b) Perforated posts of dental implants encourage alveolar bone regeneration.

136. (b) The maxillary second molar has three roots, a mesiobuccal, a distobuccal, and a lingual; second premolars have a single root. Furcation occurs in the anatomic area of a multirooted tooth when the roots divide. Furcation involvement relates to bone loss in the presence of bifurcation or trifurcation.

137. (a) The presence of plaque contributes to the development of both caries and periodontal disease.

138. (b) Plaque starts to form immediately after food ingestion and takes about 24 hours to form again after complete removal.

139. (d) Color changes are observed as vascularization changes or as venous stasis occurs, starting in the interdental papillae and gingival margin.

140. (b) Patients with acute necrotizing ulcerative gingivitis also have a general feeling of illness and rapid destruction of marginal and interproximal soft tissue.

141. (b) Stress, fatigue, and a poor diet are other factors contributing to acute necrotizing ulcerative gingivitis.

142. (b) (d) (a) (e) Gingivitis is characterized by the typical signs of inflammation, swelling, redness, pain, increased heat, and sometimes a disturbance of function.

143. (d) The other features listed in the question are characteristic of an *infrabony* pocket.

144. (b) A lingual pack is joined at the distal surface of the last tooth to the facial pack. The strips are joined interproximally by applying gentle pressure on the facial and lingual surfaces. The pack should cover the gingiva, but extension onto uninvolved tissue should be avoided, and a curette may be used to fasten the dressing around the teeth.

145. (c) Plaque control is essential to curb root sensitivity. Consideration of the use of antisensitivity preparations may be advised for patients to apply at home. Sensitivity results when dentin is exposed and should slowly disappear after a few weeks.

146. (d) A periodontal probe measures the depth of the sulcus, examines the gingiva for bleeding (the most important sign of inflammation), and determines the tissue characteristics of the pocket. It also may be used to assess the quantity of supragingival calculus on the lingual surface of the six mandibular anterior teeth.

147. (b) After a probe is inserted subgingivally, it is kept within the sulcus and the tip is walked along the junctional epithelium. The oral cavity is divided into sextants from tooth #1 through #32. Measurements are recorded at six points on each tooth: three from the buccal (distobuccal, buccal, and mesiobuccal) and three from the lingual (distolingual, lingual, and mesiolingual).

148. (c) Class II and III furcations at the roots of teeth are *not* a contraindication to using an ultrasonic scaler for removing excess cement on the coronal surface of the teeth.

149. (a) Morse scalers are designed to adapt for removing calculus and for root planing on thin roots and narrow pockets.

150. (c) In regard to mobility, 0 = normal; 1 = slight; 2 = moderate, 1 mm displacement; and 3 = extreme, more than 1 mm in all directions.

151. (a) Coronal polishing is used to remove extrinsic stains and before placement of a rubber dam.

152. (d) Intrinsic stains are not removed from the teeth by polishing with abrasive agents.

153. (a) A porte polisher may be used on teeth hypersensitive to the heat generated by rubber cup polishings. The porte polisher is also useful for polishing tooth surfaces that are difficult to reach with a prophylaxis angle; also, it is frequently used where dental facilities are limited.

154. (c) The normal depth of the gingival sulcus is 3 mm.

155. (a) (d) (e) (g) (h) (j) (k) (l)

156. (c) Topical application of fluorides does not neutralize the pH of plaque formation.

157. (a) Application of calcium hydroxide, a common procedure when permanent pulp is involved, often produces acute pulpal inflammation in primary teeth.

158. (d) Application of a sealant may depend on whether the tooth has been erupted less than 4 years, whether a patient is receiving other preventive treatment, and whether a patient has a positive history of previous occlusal lesions of the teeth.

159. (c) Luxation is applied to compress the bone cells within the tooth socket and enlarge the socket before extraction. The force is applied to the tooth using forceps.

160. (b) Surgical removal of the cordlike formation separating the maxillary centrals is referred to as a *frenectomy*.

161. (c) To prevent unraveling of the knot of the suture after surgery, the extension of the suture material is left 2 to 3 mm beyond the knot.

162. (d) For a patient's safety, the number of sutures placed must be recorded on the patient's chart to make sure all sutures are removed. Sutures remaining in the tissues interfere with healing.

163. (c) Exfoliative cytologic evaluation uses exfoliated soft-tissue cells from the tongue, cheeks, or mucosa for diagnostic purposes. The lesion is cleansed by irrigation with a mild saline solution, and the surface is scraped with a sterile wooden tongue blade.

164. (b) Class IV cytologic findings strongly suggest a malignancy.

165. (d) Before extraction, a periosteotome is used to detach the gingival tissue from around the cervix of a tooth to prevent tearing of the periosteum.

166. (b) To reduce serum cholesterol levels, polyunsaturated and monounsaturated fats are recommended. They are of vegetable origin, *not* animal fat.

167. (c) Complex carbohydrates, green leafy vegetables, citrus fruits, and bananas are recommended for dental patients with cardiovascular diseases.

168. (b) Counseling a patient about diet, caries prevention, and the control of dental plaque is important. Patients are resistant to radical reform of their dietary habits, and it is unrealistic to expect a person to abstain permanently from all cariogenic foods.

169. (b) Postextraction patients need nutritious but soft diets including foods such as cooked cereal, rice, applesauce, milk, and juices.

170. (d) When counseling dental patients about their diet, cultural background, food habits, basic nutrition, economic status, and physical condition must be taken into consideration.

171. 1: (c) (f) ; 2: (a) (f) ; 3: (d) (e) ; 4: (b) (e) (g)

Vitamin A is important for growth, health of the eyes, and cell structure and function. It promotes health of the oral structures. The B vitamins function as coenzymes, and a deficiency of one impairs the utilization of the other. Complete metabolism of carbohydrates depends on the presence of adequate amounts of each of the B complex vitamins. Vitamin C is essential to the formation and maintenance of capillary walls, and to healing. It is important to the health of the gums. Calcium functions in the development and maintenance of bones and teeth, the clotting of blood, and normal muscle activity.

172. (d) Physical complications such as respiratory tract infection and emphysema, difficulty in communication, and emotional instability can greatly hamper patients' ability to follow instructions and are contraindications to the use of relative analgesia.

173. (c) The advantages of using relative analgesia to relax an anxious patient include the ease of administration, an alert and cooperative patient, and rapid recovery when the nitrous oxide–oxygen is turned off. After administration of gases, patients feel relaxed and rested.

174. (d) After the nitrous oxide and oxygen tanks are checked for contents and pressure, the tanks are checked for operation, the air vent on the mask is closed, the exhaust valve is open, the patient is administered 5 to 8 liters of 100 percent oxygen for 1 minute, oxygen is decreased 1 liter per minute, and nitrous oxide is increased 1 liter per minute until the patient's baseline is reached.

175. (a) If patients snort when receiving nitrous oxide–oxygen, they are breathing too deeply, thus causing the mask to seal at the nostrils. If they exhale too strongly through the mask, the vent valve makes a whistling sound.

176. (d) If a patient becomes nauseous during administration of nitrous oxide–oxygen, the assistant (under direct supervision of the dentist) immediately turns off the nitrous oxide valve, turns the oxygen control to 100 percent, and slightly elevates the patient's head.

177. (b) On completion of a procedure for a patient who has received nitrous oxide–oxygen, the valves of the unit are adjusted as follows: nitrous oxide to 0 and oxygen to 100 percent. After 4 to 5 minutes on 100 percent oxygen, the patient is checked for comfort and dismissed.

178. (c) Visible light–cured impression materials have the advantage of requiring no mixing and have a more flexible working time because they do not set until they are exposed to visible light.

179. a: ② ③ ; b: ⑤ ; c: ① ④ ; d: ⑥

The amount of water used in the mix affects the strength and hardness of the product. The amount used should be just sufficient to fill the spaces between particles and to produce the first lubricating film between them. Too little water causes a dry, crumbly mass. Higher than normal water temperature accelerates setting time; the longer and more rapid the mixing, the more rapid the set.

180. (a) In the lost-wax technique, gypsum-bonded investment material expands without fracturing when heated in the burn-out oven and compensates for the shrinkage of the casting when cooling.

181. (a) A porcelain-fused-to-metal crown is one that has a recessed area on the facial surface to receive a veneer. A porcelain veneer is prepared to be baked onto the metal crown (precious metal).

182. (b) The resin dough is placed in the area of the prepared tooth within the initial alginate impression, and the impression is reseated in the patient's mouth for about 3 minutes when initial set of the resin has occurred.

183. (b) After cementation of a cast crown, using an explorer, excess cement is removed before final set of the cement; caution is used to avoid scratching the surface of the casting with the explorer.

184. (c) A mix for an insulating base should be of a thick, puttylike consistency. Of the instruments listed in the question, a spoon excavator would be the least likely used.

185. (c) To cover and protect the pulpal area and allow adequate space for restorative material, a maximum of 0.50 to 0.75 mm of insulative base may be used.

186. (e) The basic use of zinc oxide–eugenol cement is insulative. It is effective in protecting a sensitive pulp from thermal shock, and sets rapidly when in contact with saliva.

187. (a) The key punch hole, or anchor tooth hole, is the hole put over the tooth holding the clamp. Facial and lingual punch holes are made 2 to 2.5 mm distal to the anterior abutment punch hole to secure the rubber dam system to the solder point with the use of dental floss.

188. ⓓ There are five punch hole sizes on a rubber dam punch plate. Number 2, the smallest hole, is indicated for mandibular anteriors; number 5 is for large mandibular or maxillary molars and fixed bridges.

189. ⓓ The four-number instrument formula identifies the numbers as follows (left to right): The first number describes the width of the blade in tenths of a millimeter; the second number indicates the angle formed by the cutting edge and axis of the instrument handle in degrees of a centrigrade circle (this is the correct answer to the question); the third number is the length of the blade in millimeters; and the fourth number describes the angle and the long axis of the handle in degrees of a centigrade circle.

190. ⓑ Disuse atrophy occurs when a tooth loses function and the periodontal ligament shrinks.

191. ⓒ To stabilize a rubber dam that involves a fixed bridge, dental tape is threaded around a solder joint. Special holes are punched in the rubber dam to accommodate this.

192. ⓑ Ferrier separators are used to achieve mesial/distal separation on the occlusal surfaces of the teeth to prevent the separator from sliding up the roots as force is applied. The bows may be stabilized with compound.

193. ⓐ Elliptical burs have a reverse taper and are also known as *elongated round burs*. A pear-shaped bur is a classic example of this type of bur.

194. ⓒ This light system illuminates the bur and working area. A fiber-optic light projects a dual beam of light from the head of the handpiece and is activated by the fast rheostat.

195. ⓓ ⓐ ⓕ ⓑ ⓔ ⓒ Black's steps for a cavity preparation form the approach to removing caries from a tooth and preparing it for a restoration.

196. ⓓ A dentist may opt to forego the use of cotton rolls in the maxillary vestibule because of the lack of salivary glands in that location. Hence, there is little moisture to contaminate the area.

197. ⓐ The four prongs of a rubber dam clamp should precisely engage a tooth at its four corners. If a prong does not engage the tooth, tension from the rubber causes it to teeter.

198. ⓒ A larger number of teeth protruding through the rubber dam provides operator access, reflects the lips, and allows a sufficient number of dry teeth to serve as finger rests. Leaving seven to eight teeth exposed also aids in maintaining stability of the dam.

199. ⓒ A right channel placement of the loop of a Tofflemire retainer is used on the lower left and upper right quadrants. This is also referred to as a *universal retainer*.

200. ⓒ ⓓ ⓐ ⓔ ⓑ ⓕ ⓖ

201. (a) Cleoid-discoid carvers are ideally shaped for refining occlusal surfaces of restorations.

202. (c) Failure of enamel to coalesce at the unions of the lobes causes fissures. Entrapment of organic elements of the enamel-forming organ results in a natural pit or thin portion of organic substance separating the lobes. When this organic material is dissolved by enzymatic and bacterial action, a natural passage into the recesses of the enamel is created.

203. a: (1); b: (3); c: (4); d: (2); e: (1); f: (4); g: (3); h: (1) (3)

204. (a) The evacuator tip of a high-velocity evacuator is placed over the tongue, lingual to the position of the handpiece to control the fluids when an operator is working on the maxillary right facial or occlusal surfaces.

205. (c) Light-cured systems for composite resins frequently are in single paste form, and the set of the material is initiated by exposure to a halogen white light for 15 to 20 seconds per tooth.

206. (b) To ensure retention of a direct composite resin, the enamel margins and dentin of the prepared tooth are etched with approximately 50 percent phosphoric acid to create retentive tags on the surfaces. The tooth is then rinsed and dried and is ready to receive the direct composite resin.

207. (b) Patients reared on a fluoridated water supply have enamel that is resistant to decalcification and often require reapplication of the acid etching procedure.

208. (d) The sequence for preparing tooth surfaces for placement of pit and fissure sealants begins with cleansing the tooth with a pumice wash abrasive. (Note: A fluoride abrasive deters adhesion of the sealant.) Enamel is etched for 15 to 30 seconds, rinsed, and dried, followed by application of the sealant on the etched enamel on each tooth surface for 20 seconds.

209. (a) Sealant can be applied and reapplied to fill the fossae evenly. If the area is overfilled, there will be interference with normal occlusion.

210. (c) The approximate placement for the end of the white curing light tube is 2 mm from the tooth surface coated with sealant.

211. (d) Retention of sealants on teeth depends on an etched surface with enamel or dentin tags. If the tooth surface is not properly etched when rinsed and dried, reapplication of the etchant material is in order. An etched tooth surface appears frosty or satiny.

212. (d) To apply an enamel sealant, a camel's hair brush is used to coat the etched enamel with sealant on the occlusal surface. The white curing light is held approximately 2 mm from the coated surface for 20 seconds. For protection, the operator and patient wear special eye wear or a shield.

213. (d) A concentration of 35 to 50 percent phosphoric acid is supplied by manufacturers in solution or gel. The acid is applied continuously and left undisturbed in contact with the enamel for a minimum of 1 minute.

214. (b) Either division may exhibit unilateral malpositioning of two or more teeth.

215. (c) If etching solution is rubbed on the enamel before direct bonding, the bonding material cannot adhere because the tags are removed. The enamel thus loses its ability to hold the resin projections.

216. (a) In orthodontic treatment, light force arch wire may be placed 5 minutes after completion of direct bonding of the brackets to the enamel.

217. (b) Instruments used for bonding bracket material may be cleaned with chloroform or acetone. Caution: Use in a well-ventilated area.

218. (a) Dried adhesive should be removed from the enamel surface using a scaler before loose bonded brackets are replaced.

219. (c) Elastic separators are seated between the contact areas with a seesaw motion and are positioned to encircle the contact area and surround it on all sides.

220. (b) After a TP spring separator has been engaged in the contact, it may be pushed into place with an index finger or blunt instrument.

221. (c) For safety and accuracy when placing the brass wire separator, more control is achieved when using a hemostat in guiding the brass wire through the contact. A hemostat also is used to grasp the ends of a pigtail and the wire and twisting them to form separation.

222. (d) A distal shoe appliance is used to maintain the space of a primary second molar that has been lost before the eruption of the permanent first molar. The appliance is fragile, and no occlusal function can be restored because of its lack of strength.

223. (a) (a) (b) (c)

224. (d) (g) (e) (a) (f) (c) (b) (h)

225. (d) Arch wires are ligated using preformed stainless steel wires placed around the four projections of the bonded bracket. The ends of the tie wire are crossed, tightly wound, and cut 2.5 to 3 mm in length. The pigtail is tucked toward the gingiva. Preformed elastic rings may also be slipped over the projections of the bonded bracket, ligating the arch wire in place.

226. (d) The exception in the instrumentation listed for a coronal polishing procedure is a contra-angle handpiece. The handpiece used for coronal polishing is a right-angle or "prophy" handpiece.

227. (c) An anatomic crown is a total crown that is partially covered with gingival tissue, and a clinical crown is the area to be treated. The slow-speed angle should be used with stroking, wiping, and lifting action, away from the gingiva.

228. ⓒ Interproximal contact areas and embrasures are cleaned with careful application of nonwaxed dental floss or tape and fine-grit polishing strips such as cuttlefish strips.

229. ⓓ With the patient's head turned to the right and the operator at the 9 o'clock position, all surfaces noted are readily accessible.

230. ⓓ If an operator is at the 11 o'clock position, the mouth mirror is placed on the anterior portion of the tongue to retract it. If the operator is at the 9 o'clock position, the mirror is placed vertically on the tongue.

231. ⓑ The thumb and first two fingers are needed to hold an instrument. The little finger is too weak, and the fourth finger maintains a fulcrum.

232. ⓒ The cup should always be directed away from the gingiva in a coronal polishing procedure, and a stroking, wiping, lifting motion should be used to prevent overheating the tooth.

233. ⓒ

234. ⓐ Fluoride definitely deters the etching process.

235. ⓐ A palliative treatment with calcium hydroxide and zinc oxide–eugenol covered with a stainless steel crown would be effective for repair of the pulp and protection of the tooth from further trauma while healing is taking place.

236. ⓒ Calcium hydroxide is placed over the pulp exposure to promote pulp healing and formation of reparative dentin. Zinc oxide–eugenol and a stainless steel crown protect the traumatized tooth while healing takes place.

237. ⓑ A bite plane is constructed of cold cure acrylic and is cemented onto the opposing anteriors. The patient occludes on the bite plane, thus guiding the tooth out of its malalignment in the arch.

238. ⓒ A stainless steel crown must fit snugly and approximately 0.05 mm beneath the free gingiva, maintain integrity in the arch, and provide contact with the occlusal and marginal ridges of the adjacent teeth in the arch.

239. ⓒ If the pulp of a traumatized tooth has recovered, rebuilding the crown could entail placing a stainless steel crown with zinc phosphate cement; a polycarbonate crown with calcium hydroxide and zinc oxide–eugenol cement or acid-etched enamel; or a composite build-up, possibly covered by a veneer or a full gold crown.

240. ⓓ An indirect pulp capping procedure is used if a carious lesion is deep and there is a danger of pulp exposure if all of the caries is removed. After placement of a layer of palliative zinc oxide–eugenol cement, zinc phosphate cement and an amalgam may be used to restore the tooth to function.

241. ⓐ ⓒ ⓔ ⓕ ⓓ ⓑ ⓖ

242. ⓐ ⓔ ⓖ ⓕ ⓓ ⓑ ⓒ ⓗ

243. ⓐ   In an instrumentation setup, round burs in a high-speed handpiece are used to remove isolated pits and refine fissures before the placement of sealants or preventive resin restorations.

244. ⓓ   Ivory clamps are commonly used in pediatric restorative dentistry.

245. ⓑ   The crown margins should be trimmed parallel to the contour of the gingival tissue and should have no straight lines or sharp angles.

246. ⓐ   Stainless steel crowns must be contoured and crimped to fit tightly. Contouring involves bending the gingival third of a crown's margins to restore anatomic features of the natural crown.

247. ⓓ   The crimped cervical margins of a stainless steel crown provide close adaptation and mechanical retention on the tooth, protect the cement from washing by oral fluids, and maintain gingival integrity and health.

248. ⓑ   Holes should be punched so that a rubber dam is centered horizontally on the face if the lesions are interproximal, at least one tooth anterior and one tooth posterior of the involved tooth.

249. ⓑ   Stannous fluoride and acidulated phosphate fluoride are most effective in creating caries-resistant enamel because they have a lower pH and react on the apatite crystal of the enamel.

250. ⓓ   If plaque is present, coronal polishing is prescribed before fluoride application. If calculus is present, a thorough prophylaxis must be performed.

251. ⓒ   A rubber dam might also be included in the list of supplies for pulpotomy.

252. ⓐ   Sodium hypochlorite helps dissolve organic material; alternative solutions are sterile saline solution and anesthetic solution.

253. ⓑ   Placing a clamped rigid mold, holding the acrylic resin with artificial teeth, into boiling water under pressure cures the resin.

254. ⓒ   Zinc phosphate is hard and strong but highly acidic and irritating to the pulp and, without the protection of a varnish or other form of base material, could produce irreparable pulpal damage. It is used to lute cast restorations or stainless steel crowns to the teeth. It also provides bulk and protects against thermal shock.

255. ⓐ   A cool, dry slab and spatula are used for first mixing a small amount of zinc phosphate cement powder into the liquid, deliberately spatulating the mix and permitting it to stand for 30 seconds to neutralize the acid in the mix.

The next step is to incorporate more powder into the mix, obtaining a suitable mix in approximately 90 seconds.

256. ⓓ The desired consistency of zinc phosphate cement is always achieved by adding more powder and never by adding new liquid to the mix. A puttylike consistency is obtained by rapidly adding powder after the slowly mixed cement has reached a creamy texture.

257. ⓑ When the cement has reached its initial set, an explorer may be used to remove the excess around the gingival margin of the tooth.

258. ⓒ A smooth, medium-viscosity mix of zinc oxide–eugenol is needed to flow into the crevices of a tooth preparation and the inner portion of the temporary coverage. Zinc acetate crystals could be incorporated into the mix to accelerate the set, not retard it.

259. 1: ⓐ; 2: ⓒ; 3: blank; 4: ⓑ; 5: blank.

Paste is placed on the conductive tip rather than on the tooth surface.

260. ⓒ The Glick #1 was developed for placement of temporary restorations with the paddle end and removal of excess gutta percha with the heater plugger end.

261. ⓒ There is no proof that chelators soften or remove canal obstructions.

262. ⓑ Percussion is tapping of a normal or a suspected tooth with the handle of a mouth mirror or similar object. The reaction of the pulp of a sensitized tooth causes distress to a patient. The dentist usually taps a tooth in the arch in the opposite quadrant for the patient to experience the procedure before tapping an affected tooth.

263. 1: ⓕ; 2: ⓐ; 3: ⓒ; 4: ⓔ; 5: ⓓ; 6: ⓖ; 7: ⓑ; 8: ⓗ

264. ⓓ A three-way syringe on the dental unit provides water only (cold or warm), compressed air, or water spray and may be used to retract the lip, cheek, or tongue.

265. ⓐ Preformed orthodontic bands are designed to adapt to each type of tooth; they also are designed for the position in the arch, maxillary or mandibular. A band is selected and placed on a cast of the patient's dentition before being cemented at chairside.

266. ⓒ The distance from the incisal edge of a banded maxillary central tooth to the bracket slot is measured with a Boone gauge and is approximately 4.5 mm.

267. ⓑ A band is first placed with finger pressure. A Schure instrument or condenser under moderate pressure is used to seat the band further on the tooth.

268. (a) Thumb sucking may cause the teeth to be extended outward from normal alignment or to be asymmetrically out of alignment, resulting in an open bite.

269. (c) The most efficient method of seating an arch wire is to carefully and simultaneously seat both ends into the tube slots on the bands of maxillary first molars.

270. (a) A custom wedge is placed from the lingual surface interproximally on the mesial or distal surface at the gingival floor of the cavity preparation. The wedge presses the custom band against the tooth structure below the contact area.

271. (a) Wood and plastic are commonly used for commercial wedges to be placed interproximally and to hold the matrix against the tooth at the embrasure. A custom wedge may be constructed using self-polymerizing acrylic.

272. (c) A matrix band for a Class II three-surface amalgam restoration is adapted snugly at the gingival margin of the preparation to provide for adequate bulk of material, to provide contacts of the mesial/distal surfaces with adjacent teeth in the arch, and to prevent excess material from being compressed beyond the gingival margin of the tooth.

273. (a) When removing an arch wire, a Schure instrument or a scaler is used to lift the pigtail from the bracket. Caution is advised to avoid injury to the gingiva.

274. (a) Schedule I drugs are usually considered over-the-counter drugs.

275. (d) Valium is a tranquilizer that helps patients to be more receptive to changes in their lives, thus more relaxed.

276. (a) Type II gypsum material includes plaster of Paris and laboratory plaster used to pour primary impressions and study casts and for mounting inter-arch bite registrations. The crystals of plaster are spongy and take up water, producing the correct consistency for a satisfactory mix in constructing study casts.

277. (b) Although varnishes have low thermal conductivity, they are not generally applied in a sufficiently thick film to provide the thickness required for thermal insulation.

278. (c) The darkened canal space in tooth 9 in the figure that accompanies the question indicates that the root has received endodontic treatment and the space is filled with gutta percha, a radiopaque material. The circle at the apex of the root indicates radiotranslucency of the alveolus following removal of an apical abscess. This rationale can be verified in a periapical radiograph of this area.

279. (a) An X is used to designate missing teeth. They may have been extracted or may not have formed initially.

280. (a) Teeth numbered 15 and 30 in the figure that precedes question 278 are restored with full gold crowns. Teeth numbered 13 and 15 are prepared with gold crowns, which serve as abutments for a three-unit bridge supporting a pontic that replaces tooth 14.

281. (b) For a tooth to be receptive to fluoride application, the enamel surface must be free of mucin, plaque, and food debris. Paste formulas used in cleaning the enamel may contain fluoride or silicone dioxide. The teeth are then rinsed with water and dried before application of fluoride gel placed in preformed trays, and a saliva ejector is used. Patients are cautioned not to swallow during the procedure.

282. (a) Eight percent stannous fluoride gel is placed on an absorbent liner in a preformed commercial tray, which is placed first on the mandibular arch and left in place for 4 to 5 minutes. The maxillary arch is treated next; however, in some cases, both trays can be seated simultaneously. A saliva ejector may be used during this procedure to remove the excess fluids.

283. (d) Leaving a fluoride application on the teeth for at least 4 minutes favors a greater fluoride reaction with the apatite crystals. Avoiding rinsing the oral cavity immediately after treatment contributes to success of the treatment.

284. (b) For safety reasons and to provide time for fluoride to be absorbed by the enamel, patients are advised not to eat or drink for at least 30 minutes after fluoride treatment.

285. (c) The final polishing of removable prostheses is accomplished using a fresh rag wheel and tripoli paste. Sanitation to avoid cross-contamination dictates the use of a fresh rag wheel. Tripoli is a very fine abrasive used to produce a highly polished smooth surface. When polishing removable prostheses, only the gingival area is polished. An exception is a surface of acrylic that fits next to the mucosa.

286. (b) Partial dentures are placed in a solution of sodium hypochlorite to remove the debris and to sanitize the prosthesis. A removable partial denture may also be placed in an ultrasonic cleaner for a few minutes for cleaning, particularly if calculus is evident.

287. (d) Sutures, when present, should be coated with petroleum jelly or glycerine prior to placement of the periodontal pack in order to prevent their sticking to the material.

288. (c) The next of kin should immediately be notified; paramedics should be called; and both the coroner's office and the state board of dentistry should be apprised of the occurrence. The patient's records should never be altered, but additional information may be appended if the date, time, and signature of the dentist are noted. Any emergency procedures taken or the physical appearance of the patient could be described in this manner for the record.

289. (d) A custom acrylic crown is contructed in an alginate impression taken before the tooth is prepared for a permanent crown. Tooth shade acrylic is placed into the impression of the tooth prepared for the crown. The acrylic crown is taken from the alginate impression, adjusted and temporarily cemented to the patient's tooth *after* the preparation and before the patient is dismissed.

290. (b) To prevent injury to the postsurgical tissues, remove the continuous suture a loop at a time; cut, grasp a loop of suture, and remove free from tissues.

TEST III

Dental Radiography

TEST III

1. X-rays are created when the high-voltage current and free electrons in the tube strike the

   ① cathode
   ② tungsten target
   ③ position indicator device (PID)
   ④ focal spot

      ⓐ 1, 3
      ⓑ 2, 4
      ⓒ 1, 2, 3
      ⓓ 4 only

2. An x-ray beam contains photons of various energies that relate to which aspect of the beam?

      ⓐ absorption
      ⓑ attenuation
      ⓒ heat
      ⓓ penetrating power

3. Bremsstrahlung (braking radiation) is produced when electrons collide with the nuclei of the target atoms, creating

      ⓐ short x-ray waves
      ⓑ secondary radiation
      ⓒ x-rays of various lengths
      ⓓ filtered radiation

4. The ability of x-ray photons to penetrate human tissues depends on which of the following?

   ① type of film used
   ② distance between source and object
   ③ density of the object penetrated
   ④ temperature of the anode

      ⓐ 1, 2
      ⓑ 1, 3
      ⓒ 2, 3
      ⓓ 2, 4

5. The ability of x-rays to remove electrons from a substance is called

      ⓐ braking radiation
      ⓑ particulate radiation
      ⓒ ionization
      ⓓ background radiation

6. The properties of x-rays that make them useful for dental radiography include their

   ① high frequency
   ② short wavelength
   ③ variety of wavelengths
   ④ long wavelength
   ⑤ low frequency
   ⑥ ability to be stopped by the structure entered

      ⓐ 1, 2
      ⓑ 1, 3
      ⓒ 2, 5, 6
      ⓓ 4, 5, 6

7. The shortest waves of the electromagnetic spectrum are measured in

      ⓐ A — angstrom units
      ⓑ kV — kilovoltage
      ⓒ mA — milliamperage
      ⓓ AC — alternating current

8. Atoms of cellular structures that have lost electrons are referred to as

      ⓐ binding energy neutrons

ⓑ ions

ⓒ nuclei

ⓓ photons

9. The types of tissues in the oral cavity result in radiographic imaging that is

① likely to be blurred

② dense

③ light gray or white

④ radiolucent

ⓐ 1, 2

ⓑ 1, 3

ⓒ 2, 3

ⓓ 3, 4

10. The harmful effects of x-irradiation on human tissue is

ⓐ immediately exhibited

ⓑ insignificant

ⓒ usually acute

ⓓ cumulative

11. The human tissue most sensitive to ionizing radiation is the

ⓐ cornea of the eye

ⓑ formative embryo

ⓒ connective tissue

ⓓ thyroid gland

12. Radiation hygiene during film exposure is demonstrated by which of the following

① use of low kilovoltage

② use of 12- to 16- inch PID

③ use of D- or E-speed film

④ collimation of the x-ray beam to 3.75 inches at a patient's face

ⓐ 1, 3

ⓑ 1, 4

ⓒ 2, 3

ⓓ 2, 3, 4

13. Proper radiation hygiene during the exposure of radiographs is demonstrated by

① adherence to the ALARA principle
② placing leaded aprons and thyroid collars on patients
③ retakes of all radiographs whose placement is doubtful
④ the operator holding films for patients who have difficulty in doing so

   ⓐ 1, 2
   ⓑ 1, 3
   ⓒ 2, 3
   ⓓ 2, 3, 4

14. Quality assurance in the practice of dental radiography includes

① x-ray equipment functioning efficiently
② the use of high-speed film
③ the use of a 90-kVp x-ray unit
④ application of a thyroid shield for most x-ray film exposures

   ⓐ 1, 3
   ⓑ 2, 4
   ⓒ 1, 2, 3
   ⓓ 1, 2, 4

15. The dental staff's exposure to ionizing radiation is detected by

   ⓐ keeping a log on the number of patients x-rayed
   ⓑ checking the number of films exposed
   ⓒ using the age-based formula to learn MPD
   ⓓ monitoring individual staff members

16. According to government guidelines, the yearly whole-body radiation dose for occupationally exposed workers must not exceed

   ⓐ 3 rems per calendar year
   ⓑ 5 rems per calendar year
   ⓒ 7 rems per calendar year
   ⓓ 10 rems per calendar year

17. Exceptions to government guidelines on permissible exposure to ionizing radiation by dental personnel relate to

① pregnant workers
② workers older than 60 years

③ workers younger than 18 years

④ workers who monitor with individual dosimeters

    ⓐ 1, 3

    ⓑ 1, 2, 3

    ⓒ 1, 3, 4

    ⓓ 2, 3, 4

18. What means should be taken to protect people in the surrounding area from secondary radiation?

① installation of glass windows so outsiders may be observed

② installation of wood panel wall shielding

③ maintenance of a low-radiation workload

④ installation of two layers of 5/8-inch sheet rock wall shielding

    ⓐ 1, 2

    ⓑ 1, 3

    ⓒ 2, 3

    ⓓ 4 only

19. Protecting dental patients from excess exposure to radiation is aided by the

① ⅝″ gypsum wallboard in the operatory

② use of a lead cervical collar

③ use of E-speed dental film

④ correct placement of the PID

    ⓐ 1, 2, 3

    ⓑ 1, 2, 4

    ⓒ 1, 3, 4

    ⓓ 2, 3, 4

20. Unique properties of x-rays include their ability to do all of the following EXCEPT

① penetrate organic matter

② produce a latent image

③ fluoresce all materials

④ produce ionization of matter

⑤ produce a spectrum of radiomagnetic radiation

    ⓐ 1, 2, 3

    ⓑ 1, 5

Continued on next page

       ⓒ 2, 3, 4

       ⓓ 3, 5

21. Kilovoltage of a dental x-ray machine is the property that

   ① affects the quantity of x-rays

   ② measures the electrical output

   ③ affects the quality of x-rays

   ④ affects the penetrating power

   ⑤ controls the number of x-ray photons available for use

       ⓐ 1, 2, 3

       ⓑ 3, 4

       ⓒ 2, 3, 4

       ⓓ 3, 4, 5

22. Raising the kilovoltage of an x-ray machine affects the x-rays produced by making them

   ① less penetrating

   ② more penetrating

   ③ of longer wavelength

   ④ of shorter wavelength

       ⓐ 1, 3

       ⓑ 2, 3

       ⓒ 2, 4

       ⓓ 4 only

23. The milliamperage setting of the x-ray machine controls the

   ① quantity of x-rays produced

   ② quantity of electrons

   ③ heat of the tungsten filament

   ④ quality of x-radiation produced

   ⑤ the electrical current that passes through the tungsten filament

       ⓐ 1, 2, 3

       ⓑ 1, 2, 3, 4

       ⓒ 1, 2, 3, 5

       ⓓ 2, 3, 4

24. What facts are used to ascertain the amount of total radiation a patient has received during a survey?

① milliamperage setting
② kilovoltage setting
③ exposure time
⑤ type of PID
    ⓐ 1, 3
    ⓑ 2, 4
    ⓒ 1, 2, 3
    ⓓ 3, 4

25. The tungsten filament in the dental x-ray tube is actually the
    ⓐ anode
    ⓑ filter
    ⓒ cathode
    ⓓ collimator

26. The function of the collimator in the tube head of the x-ray unit is to
① filter out unnecessary radiation
② act as a target for electrons
③ assist in thermionic emissions
④ limit the size of the x-ray beam
    ⓐ 1, 3
    ⓑ 2, 4
    ⓒ 1, 2, 3
    ⓓ 4 only

27. The collimator or lead diaphragm is designed
① with no opening
② with a small opening
③ to be part of the positioning device
④ to stop the short rays
    ⓐ 1 only
    ⓑ 1, 3
    ⓒ 2, 3
    ⓓ 2, 4

28. The PID placed at the end of the x-ray tube head

    ① may be round
    ② may restrict the diameter of the x-ray beam
    ③ may be rectangular
    ④ is usually pointed

    ⓐ 1, 2
    ⓑ 1, 2, 3
    ⓒ 1, 3, 4
    ⓓ 2, 3, 4

29. The extension from the tube head of the x-ray unit that directs the useful beam is referred to as the

    ⓐ PID
    ⓑ total filter
    ⓒ collimator
    ⓓ leaded aperture

30. The PID that is least effective in minimizing scatter radiation is the

    ⓐ pointed cone
    ⓑ cylinder with scatter guard
    ⓒ lead-lined cylinder
    ⓓ lead-lined rectangular device

31. In order to follow radiation hygiene regulations for their protection when producing dental radiographs, operators should NEVER

    ① stand in line with the primary beam
    ② hold the film in the patient's mouth during exposure
    ③ stand within 6 feet of the x-ray unit
    ④ stand behind the patient's head
    ⑤ remain in the operatory unless there is a lead barrier

    ⓐ 1, 2, 3
    ⓑ 1, 2, 4
    ⓒ 1, 2, 5
    ⓓ 2, 3, 4
    ⓔ 2, 3, 5

32. Radiation hygiene regulations for protection and comfort of patients during exposure of all panographic type exposures include

① draping with a leaded apron
② placing a leaded cervical collar
③ positioning the head of the unit near area of exposure
④ stabilizing the film placement with a holder
⑤ retaking any radiographs about which placement of film is questionable

    ⓐ 1, 2
    ⓑ 1, 4
    ⓒ 1, 2, 3, 4
    ⓓ 1, 2, 3, 5

33. The safest position for an operator during exposure of *anterior* dental films is

    ⓐ at a 45° angle to the opposite side of the patient's head
    ⓑ 6 feet behind the patient's head
    ⓒ behind the head of the x-ray unit
    ⓓ behind a lead barrier

34. Which of the following is true of filters found in an x-ray tube head?

① they are made of lead
② they are positioned in the tube head
③ they function to remove high-energy x-rays
④ filters required in a 90-kV machine relate to inherent and added filtration in the amount of 1.5 mm
⑤ they remove x-rays that add to patients' absorbed dose

    ⓐ 1, 2, 3
    ⓑ 2, 3, 5
    ⓒ 2, 4, 5
    ⓓ 2, 5

35. The safest position for an operator during exposure of films on *posterior* teeth when no lead barrier is present is

    ⓐ at a 45° angle to the opposite side of a patient's head
    ⓑ 6 feet behind a patient's head
    ⓒ 6 feet behind the tube head
    ⓓ behind the head of the x-ray unit

36. Which of the following applies when establishing a quality assurance policy for manual radiographic processing?

Continued on next page

① weekly check of processing solutions for their strength and quality
② processing exposed film using standard time and temperature
③ exposing film using a metallic step wedge
④ replenishing developer with water when necessary to maintain level

  ⓐ 1, 2
  ⓑ 1, 3
  ⓒ 2, 3
  ⓓ 2, 4

37. Standard requirements for a darkroom for manual processing of exposed films include

① a facility with dark-colored walls
② hot and cold running water with mixing valves
③ sources of white light and a safelight
④ a dryer equipped with a fan
⑤ an accurate thermometer in the tank

  ⓐ 1, 2, 3
  ⓑ 1, 4
  ⓒ 2, 3
  ⓓ 2, 3, 5

38. Which of the following applies to automatic film processors?

① total processing time is reduced
② glutaraldehyde is added to the developer to prevent softening of the emulsion
③ processing solutions are kept warmer than for manual processing
④ rollers should be cleaned weekly
⑤ processed film is dried in a separate dryer

  ⓐ 1, 2
  ⓑ 1, 3
  ⓒ 2, 3, 4
  ⓓ 2, 3, 5

39. Which of the following could cause a processed radiograph to be too light?

① exhausted developer
② fixing time too short
③ developing time too short

④ cold processing solutions

⑤ failure to circulate rinsing bath

     ⓐ 1, 2, 3

     ⓑ 1, 3, 4

     ⓒ 1, 3, 5

     ⓓ 2, 4, 5

40. If processed dental films are yellow or brown, the cause is

① exhausted developer

② exhausted fixer

③ incomplete fixing

④ insufficient washing

⑤ defective safelight

     ⓐ 1, 2, 3

     ⓑ 1, 2, 4

     ⓒ 1, 3, 4

     ⓓ 2, 3, 5

     ⓔ 3, 4, 5

41. Which of the following has occurred when spots appear on processed radiographs?

① premature contact with fixer

② water droplets on film before processing

③ premature contact with developer

④ static electricity when film pack is opened

⑤ processing solutions too warm

     ⓐ 1, 3

     ⓑ 1, 2, 3

     ⓒ 2, 3, 4

     ⓓ 2, 3, 5

42. Extremely dense radiographs may result from which of the following?

① remaining in the fixer too long

② remaining in the developer too long

③ temperature of solutions too high

④ varying thickness of the alveolus

⑤ insufficient exposure time

Continued on next page

(a) 1, 2
(b) 1, 2, 3
(c) 1, 4, 5
(d) 2, 3, 4
(e) 2, 4, 5

43. Fogged film may be the result of which of the following?

① white light leaks in the darkroom
② defective safelights
③ exposure of film to unwanted radiation
④ exposure of film to the safelight before fixing is completed
⑤ placing the film in the mouth backward

(a) 1, 2, 3
(b) 1, 3, 4
(c) 2, 3, 4
(d) 3, 4, 5

44. When using conventional processing solutions, the wet dental film may be safely viewed

① after a maximum of 2 minutes in the fixer
② after a minimum of 3 minutes in the fixer
③ after the film is rinsed in running water
④ only under the darkroom safelight

(a) 1, 3
(b) 2, 3
(c) 2, 4
(d) 2, 3, 4

45. The error exhibited by a maxillary premolar film with a mesial cone cut and a clear image of the second premolar and the first and second molars is

(a) film placement too posterior
(b) PID placement too posterior
(c) PID placement too anterior
(d) film placement too anterior

46. The proper procedure for mounting a complete dental radiographic survey includes which of the following?

① notation of the patient's name, the date when films were exposed, and the name of the prescribing dentist

② the use of an opaque film mount with unused spaces blocked out

③ mounting individual radiographs in anatomic order

④ placing periapical and bitewing radiographs in the same mount

⑤ noting total exposure time

    ⓐ 1, 2

    ⓑ 1, 2, 3, 4

    ⓒ 2, 3, 4, 5

    ⓓ 2, 4, 5

47. What is the cause when only one or two films of a complete dental survey are clear after being processed?

    ⓐ cold processing solutions

    ⓑ overexposure

    ⓒ no exposure

    ⓓ incorrect processing

    ⓔ partial exposure

48. The type or size darkroom safelight selected may be

① 7 watts

② 15 watts

③ dependent on type of film to be processed

④ dependent on the type or amount of filtration

    ⓐ 1, 3

    ⓑ 2, 4

    ⓒ 1, 2, 3

    ⓓ all of the above

49. The height of the safelight above the darkroom bench should be at least

    ⓐ 4 feet

    ⓑ 5 feet

    ⓒ 6 feet

    ⓓ 7 feet

50. Flaws or faults exhibited in the production of intraoral radiographs are due to what types of errors?

    ⓐ exposure errors

    ⓑ processing errors

    ⓒ film handling

Continued on next page

(d) film storage

(e) all of the above

51. An x-ray tube is composed of a sealed glass envelope and

① an anode

② a filter

③ a cathode

④ a focusing cup

⑤ a collimator

(a) 1, 2, 3

(b) 1, 3, 4

(c) 2, 3

(d) 2, 4, 5

(e) all of the above

52. From what portion of the negative pole of the x-ray tube are electrons emitted?

(a) tungsten filament

(b) tungsten target

(c) focal spot

(d) copper stem

53. The quality or penetrating ability of the electrons is controlled by the setting of the

(a) kilovoltage meter

(b) milliamperage meter

(c) electronic timer

(d) copper stem

54. Considering evaporation and use, the developer in a manual processor should be replenished at a rate of a

(a) minimum of 4 to 5 ounces daily

(b) minimum of 6 to 8 ounces daily

(c) maximum of 10 ounces daily

(d) maximum of 12 ounces daily

55. The correct replenishment rate for automatic roller-type processors containing 1 gallon each of developer and fixer is

(a) 6 ounces daily

(b) 8 ounces daily

(c) 10 ounces daily

(d) 12 ounces daily

56. When considering the desired contrast of components of a radiograph, the reference is to the

(a) lightness and whiteness

(b) radiopacity and radiolucency

(c) darkness or blackness

(d) shades of gray

57. The total number of x-rays emitted from the focal spot of the tube head is expressed in

(a) rads

(b) kVs

(c) mAs

(d) rems

58. The beam of x-rays that leaves the target is composed of what type of rays?

① short wavelength

② long wavelength

③ penetrating

④ hard rays

⑤ soft rays

(a) 1, 2, 3

(b) 1, 3, 4

(c) 1, 3, 5

(d) 2, 3, 5

59. When comparing the recommended exposure of E-speed film with D-speed film, the E film requires a reduction of radiation exposure by

(a) 1/4

(b) 1/2

(c) 1/3

(d) 3/8

60. During film placement, the embossed dot of the film packet should be placed toward the occlusal or incisal edges with the exception of what exposures?

   (a) maxillary molars

   (b) mandibular molars

   (c) mandibular incisors

   (d) maxillary incisors

   (e) bitewings

61. Using the parallel technique for correct vertical angulation, the opening of the PID should be positioned

   (a) perpendicular to the long axis of the teeth to be radiographed

   (b) parallel to the teeth being exposed

   (c) horizontal to the film

   (d) always at a 48° angle to the film

62. In correct horizontal angulation, the central beam is directed

   (a) at the apical third of the roots

   (b) distal to the contact areas of two adjacent teeth

   (c) through the contact areas of two adjacent teeth

   (d) on the long axis of the teeth

63. Subject contrast of a radiograph can be decreased by using a

   (1) higher milliamperage setting

   (2) higher kilovoltage setting

   (3) lower exposure time

   (4) higher exposure time

   (a) 1, 2

   (b) 1, 3

   (c) 2 only

   (d) 4 only

64. If a film packet is positioned backward in the oral cavity, the resulting radiograph will

   (1) be lighter than optimum

   (2) be darker than optimum

   (3) have a herringbone effect

   (4) exhibit routine landmarks for mounting

(a) 1, 2
(b) 1, 3
(c) 2, 3
(d) 2, 4

65. When the teeth are normally aligned and a mandibular molar film shows closed contacts with the distal part of the second premolar overlapping, the horizontal angulation should be adjusted

(a) slightly mesially
(b) slightly distally
(c) higher at the contact area
(d) lower at the contact area

66. For correct horizontal angulation, the central beam of the tube head is positioned

(a) at the occlusal contact of the teeth
(b) at right angles to the contact areas
(c) in a plus angulation
(d) distal to the contact areas

67. In intraoral radiography, film blurring is caused by movement of the

① tube head
② film
③ patient
④ PID

(a) 1, 2
(b) 1, 3
(c) 1, 4
(d) 2, 3

68. If teeth appear foreshortened on the original radiograph, the vertical angulation of the central beam for the retake is

(a) increased
(b) decreased
(c) moved mesially
(d) moved distally

69. If the cuspid appears to overlap the first premolar in a radiograph of the premolars, the horizontal angulation of the central beam in a retake is

    (a) adjusted mesially

    (b) adjusted distally

    (c) raised on the apices

    (d) moved toward the occlusal surfaces

70. To project the horizontal angulation for molar bitewings, the PID is directed through the contact between the

    (a) maxillary second premolars

    (b) first and second maxillary molars

    (c) first and second mandibular molars

    (d) mandibular second and third molars

71. Which of the following is true in regard to the paralleling technique for projection of the mandibular central incisor region?

    (1) all four incisors can be imaged on a #1 film

    (2) contact of the centrals and laterals is opened

    (3) the film remains 1 mm above the floor of the mouth

    (4) the film is placed as far into the oral cavity as possible

        (a) 1, 2

        (b) 1, 3

        (c) 1, 4

        (d) 2, 4

72. To expose a radiograph of the entire third molar region, the technique used is to direct horizontal angulation

    (a) at a distal oblique angle

    (b) at the center of the third molar

    (c) at the temporomandibular joint

    (d) at the contact between the second and third molars

73. The bisecting of the angle technique in dental radiography adapts the principle of

    (a) directing the central beam to the coronal area of the tooth

    (b) bisecting an imaginary angle formed by the plane of the film and the incline of the tooth and roots

    (c) directing the central beam to the apices of the tooth

    (d) placing the film as close to a tooth as possible

74. Occlusal dental radiographs are used to

    (a) identify caries activity

    (b) diagnose periodontal conditions

    (c) localize foreign bodies

    (d) examine lesions of the mucosa

    (e) all of the above

75. Which of the following is correct when completing an occlusal radiograph of the maxillary arch?

    (1) always place the long dimension of the film across the mouth

    (2) direct the central ray toward the bridge of the nose

    (3) use a positive vertical angulation

    (4) elevate the patient's chin

        (a) 1, 2

        (b) 1, 3

        (c) 2, 3

        (d) 2, 4

76. All of the following are causes of radiographs of poor density EXCEPT failure to

    (a) correctly evaluate a patient's bone structure

    (b) select the correct exposure factors

    (c) fully develop the exposed films

    (d) allow the films to remain in the fixing solution both before and after a wet reading

77. Which of the following is true in regard to an edentulous radiographic survey?

    (a) a typical survey may contain as many as 14 periapical films

    (b) if there is no visible evidence of pathology, radiographs should not be made

    (c) a typical survey may contain 10 perapical films and 4 bitewing films

    (d) the exposure factor should be increased by approximately as much as one-fourth the normal time

78. Failure to show the apices of the teeth in a maxillary radiograph can be caused by

    (1) failure to place the film high enough toward the palate

    (2) placing the film too close to the teeth

Continued on next page

③ insufficient vertical angulation

④ failure to place the film at an angle

ⓐ 1, 2

ⓑ 1, 3

ⓒ 2, 3

ⓓ 2, 4

79. Compared with x-rays produced by a 70-kV dental x-ray machine, x-rays produced by a 90-kV machine are

ⓐ more numerous

ⓑ of a longer wavelength

ⓒ more penetrating

ⓓ easier to filter out

80. Which one of the following occurs during the fixation aspect of film processing?

ⓐ undeveloped crystals are developed

ⓑ energized crystals are fixed

ⓒ nonenergized crystals are fixed

ⓓ silver halide crystals are precipitated into the emulsion

81. Optimum developing time and temperature for manual processing are

ⓐ 3 minutes at 72°F

ⓑ 4 minutes at 70°F

ⓒ 4.5 to 5 minutes at 68°F

ⓓ 5.0 to 5.5 minutes at 66°F

82. Which of the following is the correct technique when placing bitewing films?

ⓐ place the film as close to the teeth as possible

ⓑ bend the anterior inferior corner of the film for a patient's comfort

ⓒ keep a finger between the film and the alveolus

ⓓ tilt the inferior portion of the film toward the center of the mouth

83. Which of the following is true when exposing panoramic film?

① a thyroid collar is routinely used

② the midsagittal plane of a patient's face should be perpendicular to the floor

③ patients must stand or sit in an erect position

④ patients should place their tongue against their palate

⑤ a lead apron should be placed above the patient's clavicles

   ⓐ 1, 2, 3

   ⓑ 1, 3, 5

   ⓒ 2, 3, 4

   ⓓ 2, 3, 5

84. Film exposure time is affected by all of the following EXCEPT

① milliamperage used

② type of PID used

③ radiographic technique

④ collimator opening

⑤ target film distance

   ⓐ 1, 2, 3

   ⓑ 1, 3, 4

   ⓒ 1, 3, 5

   ⓓ 2, 4

   ⓔ 2, 5

85. According to federal regulations, the beam size should not exceed what number of inches at the patient's skin surface?

   ⓐ 1 3/4

   ⓑ 2 1/4

   ⓒ 2 3/4

   ⓓ 3

86. Which one of the following is responsible for all collimation?

   ⓐ inherent and added filters

   ⓑ tungsten target

   ⓒ lead diaphragm

   ⓓ plastic cone

87. Film contrast is dependent on which of the following?

① type of film

② density of the subject of radiation

③ film processing

Continued on next page

④ film density

⑤ thickness of the subject of radiation

    ⓐ 1, 2, 3

    ⓑ 1, 3 4

    ⓒ 2, 3, 4

    ⓓ 2, 4, 5

88. White marks on processed panoramic radiographs may be caused by

① torn emulsion

② static electricity

③ finger contaminated with developer

④ finger contaminated with fixer

⑤ finger contaminated with stannous fluoride

    ⓐ 1, 2, 3

    ⓑ 1, 4

    ⓒ 1, 3, 5

    ⓓ 2, 3, 5

    ⓔ 3, 5

89. Which of the following is true of the paralleling periapical technique in dental radiography?

① it is used to minimize shape distortion of the radiographic image

② films should be placed parallel to the crowns of the teeth

③ the central ray is aimed perpendicular to the film and the long axis of the tooth

④ film-holding devices are not necessary

    ⓐ 1, 2

    ⓑ 1, 3

    ⓒ 2, 3

    ⓓ 2, 4

90. Which of the following are true in regard to the edentulous radiographic technique?

① bisecting the angle technique should be used

② the distortion inherent in the bisecting the angle technique does not interfere with diagnosis of infrabony conditions

③ exposure time should be reduced by about one-fourth the normal time

④ use of bisecting the angle technique reduces the amount of radiation received by patients

(a) 1, 2
(b) 1, 3
(c) 2, 3
(d) 2, 4

91. A diagnostic endodontic radiograph should ensure that
  ① the periodontal ligament is distinct
  ② the tooth is centered on the film
  ③ at least 5 mm of bone beyond the apex is visible
  ④ accessory canals are visible
  ⑤ the image is as anatomically correct as possible

   (a) 1, 2, 3
   (b) 1, 2, 4
   (c) 2, 3, 4
   (d) 2, 3, 5

92. Which of the following is an advantage of using intensifying screens when making extraoral radiographs?
  ① fewer x-rays are needed
  ② detail is enhanced
  ③ film movement during exposure is prevented
  ④ exposure time is reduced

   (a) 1, 2
   (b) 1, 3
   (c) 1, 4
   (d) 2, 3
   (e) 2, 4

93. Particles of dust on intensifying screens result in what artifacts on the film?
   (a) areas of greater density
   (b) areas of less density
   (c) scratches on film emulsion
   (d) white spots

94. Which of the following is true in regard to the care of intensifying screens?
   (a) they should be vigorously cleaned periodically with detergent
   (b) they should be cleaned periodically with a product containing an anti-static compound

Continued on next page

ⓒ the cassettes should be closed immediately after the screens are cleaned

ⓓ fingernail scratches are easily smoothed out

95. Which of the following are true of duplicating film?
① exposure to light makes them lighter
② exposure to light darkens them
③ emulsion is on one side only
④ emulsion reaction resembles that of radiographic film

    ⓐ 1 only
    ⓑ 1, 3
    ⓒ 2, 3
    ⓓ 2, 4

96. Which of the following statements is true?

    ⓐ patients' exposure to radiation should be determined by a rigid schedule
    ⓑ if a patient has recently been exposed to radiation, it is best to provide dental care without first taking diagnostic radiographs
    ⓒ before exposing any patient to ionizing radiation, documented informed consent must be obtained
    ⓓ for informed consent, patients must sign a dated consent form

97. Which of the following is true?
① radiographs are an integral part of a patient's record
② the clinician has primary property rights to a patient's records
③ patients have the right to have their radiographs forwarded to other professionals
④ the clinician must retain duplicates of all patients' records

    ⓐ 1, 2
    ⓑ 1, 3
    ⓒ 2, 4
    ⓓ 3, 4

98. Which of the following is true in regard to the duplication of films?
    (a) duplication may be performed in the operatory or laboratory
    (b) duplicating film is placed on the duplicator with the emulsion side up
    (c) radiographs are placed on the duplicator
    (d) the emulsion side of the duplicating film must be in contact with the radiographs

99. A radiographic mounting holder (x-ray mount) is illustrated below. Note that the embossed dot is raised toward the operator; identify the radiograph to be mounted in each space.

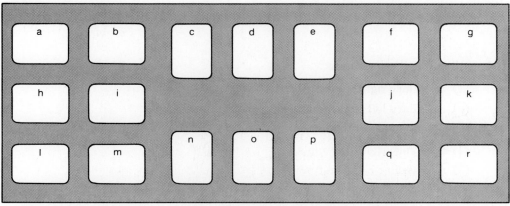

(From Torres H, Mazzuchi LE: Review of Dental Assisting. Philadelphia, WB Saunders, 1983, p 245)

Place your answer in the space provided:
a. _____   j. _____
b. _____   k. _____
c. _____   l. _____
d. _____   m. _____
e. _____   n. _____
f. _____   o. _____
g. _____   p. _____
h. _____   q. _____
i. _____   r. _____

Questions 100 through 103 are based on the radiographic survey of adult dentition shown below.

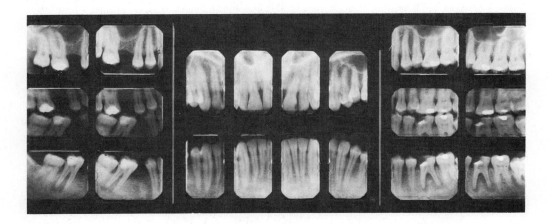

100. Which teeth are missing?

   ① maxillary right second premolar   ⓐ 1, 2

   ② maxillary left first molar   ⓑ 1, 4

   ③ mandibular left first molar   ⓒ 2, 5

   ④ maxillary right first molar   ⓓ 4, 5

   ⑤ mandibular right first molar

101. What tooth has an occlusal filling?

   ⓐ maxillary right second premolar   ⓒ mandibular left second premolar

   ⓑ maxillary left second premolar   ⓓ mandibular left second molar

102. On which radiograph are the contact areas between the maxillary premolars the most clearly open?

   ⓐ maxillary left periapical premolar   ⓒ left premolar bitewing

   ⓑ maxillary right periapical premolar   ⓓ right premolar bitewing

103. On which tooth is a portion of a crown missing?

   ⓐ mandibular right first molar   ⓒ maxillary right first molar

   ⓑ mandibular left first molar   ⓓ maxillary left first molar

Questions 104 through 106 are based on the complete radiographic survey of mixed dentition shown below.

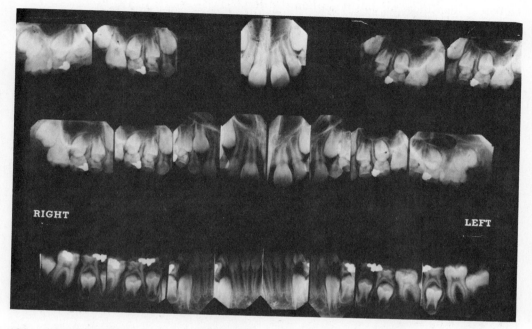

RIGHT   LEFT

104. The approximate age of the patient shown in the radiographic survey is

    (a) 5 to 7 years

    (b) 7 to 9 years

    (c) 10 to 12 years

    (d) 12 years

105. The conditions shown in the survey include

    (1) fillings in both permanent and primary teeth

    (2) impacted teeth

    (3) mixed dentition

    (4) supernumerary teeth

        (a) 1, 2

        (b) 1, 3

        (c) 2, 3

        (d) 2, 4

106. What permanent teeth are shown to be erupted?

    (a) mandibular second molars

    (b) maxillary cuspids

    (c) maxillary first molars

    (d) mandibular first premolars

The radiographs in questions 107 through 125 were exposed on a teaching manikin and on a dental patient. The position for mounting is looking at the manufacturer's embossed identification dot (bump) on the film.

107. Exposure errors exhibited in the *right premolar* bitewing shown below are caused by

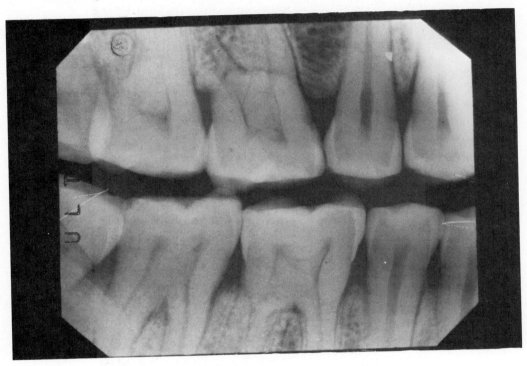

   ① PID placement too mesial
   ② PID placement too distal
   ③ negative vertical angulation
   ④ film placement too distal

      ⓐ 1, 3
      ⓑ 2, 4
      ⓒ 1, 2, 3
      ⓓ 4 only

108. Errors exhibited in the radiograph of the *mandibular right cuspid* shown below include

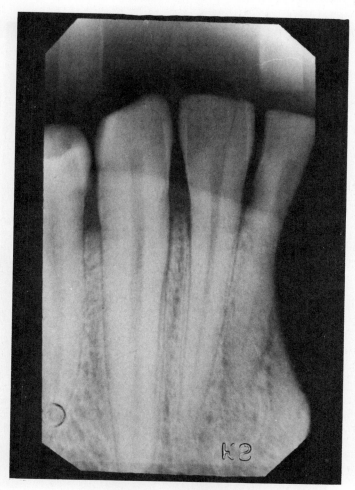

① inadequate vertical angulation
② PID placement too high
③ PID placement too low
④ processing artifact

ⓐ 1, 3
ⓑ 2, 3
ⓒ 2, 4
ⓓ 1, 3, 4

109. Errors exhibited in the radiograph of the *maxillary right cuspid* shown below include

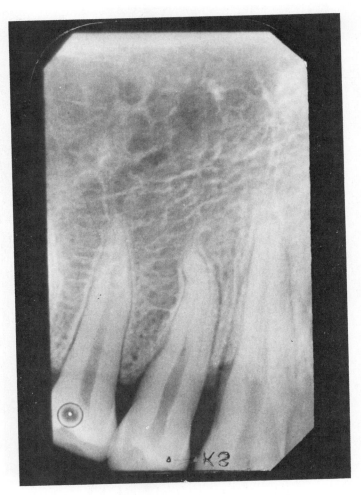

① PID placement too low
② excessive negative vertical angulation
③ excessive positive vertical angulation
④ improper film placement

    ⓐ 1, 3
    ⓑ 2, 4
    ⓒ 3, 4
    ⓓ 4 only

110. The artifact in the radiograph of the *maxillary right cuspid* shown in question 109 is due to

    ⓐ excess bending
    ⓑ cone cut

    ⓒ film placed backward

    ⓓ identification mark

111. Which of the following is evident in the *left molar bitewing* shown below?

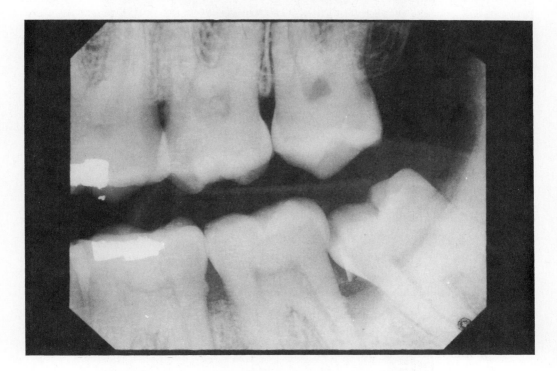

  ① horizontal angulation is too distal

  ② occlusal contacts are open in position

  ③ film placement is too mesial

  ④ vertical angulation is excessive

      ⓐ 1, 2

      ⓑ 1, 3

      ⓒ 2, 3

      ⓓ 2, 4

112. Errors exhibited in the following radiograph of the *mandibular right premolars* include

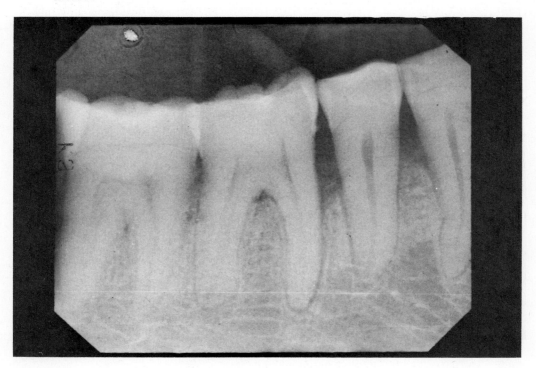

   ① film placed too distally
   ② film reversed in the mouth
   ③ fogging at distal
   ④ PID placement too distal

       ⓐ 1, 3
       ⓑ 2, 4
       ⓒ 1, 2, 3
       ⓓ 4 only

113. The error exhibited in the *right molar bitewing* shown below is

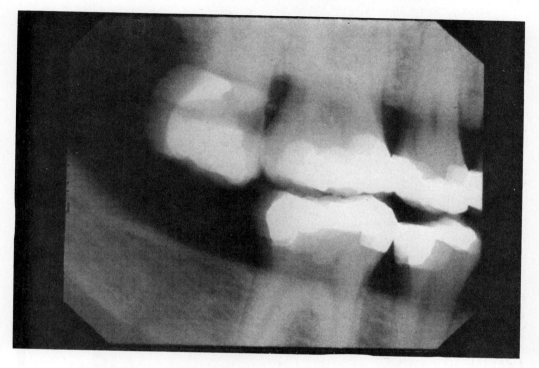

(a) excess bending of the film
(b) insufficient development
(c) patient movement
(d) tube head movement

114. The error exhibited in the automatically processed radiograph of the *mandibular left molars* shown below is due to

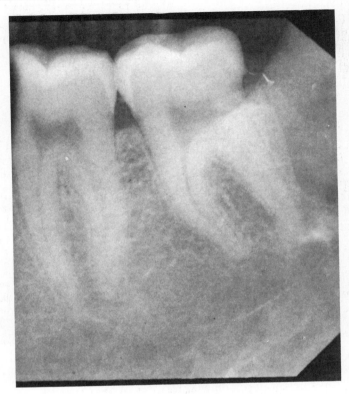

ⓐ darkroom light exposure
ⓑ film overlap
ⓒ splash marks
ⓓ insufficient development

115. The artifact exhibited in the manually processed radiograph of the *maxillary left premolars* shown below is due to

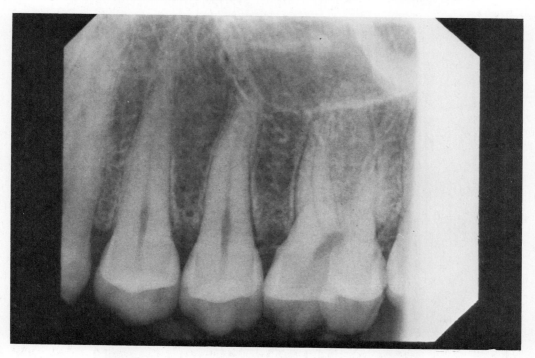

    ⓐ incorrect placement of the PID
    ⓑ level of developer solution too low
    ⓒ overlapping of film during processing
    ⓓ level of fixing solution too low

116. The errors exhibited by the manually processed radiograph of the *mandibular left premolars* shown below is due to

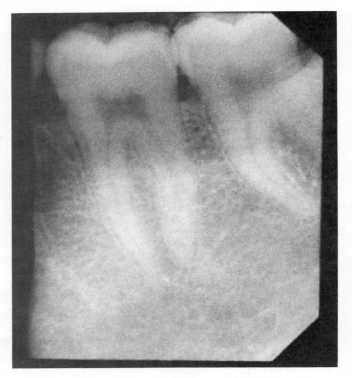

1. double exposure
2. film placement too distal
3. level of the developing solution too low
4. film placement too deep in the lingual vault

    (a) 1, 2
    (b) 1, 3
    (c) 2, 3
    (d) 2, 4

117. The artifacts exhibited in the following radiograph of the *maxillary left premolars* that was manually processed are due to

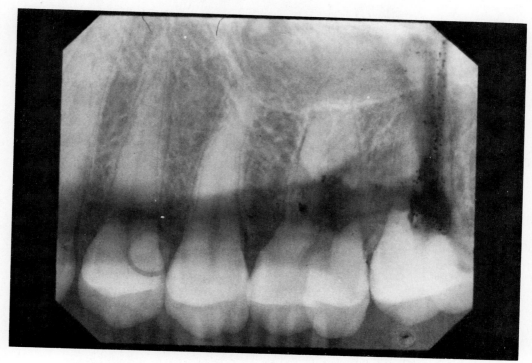

ⓐ excessive developing time
ⓑ exhausted developer solution
ⓒ double film processed as one
ⓓ dirty processing solutions

118. The artifact exhibited by the *left premolar bitewing* shown below is due to

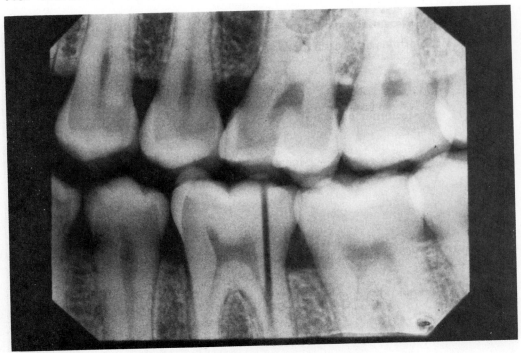

     ⓐ patient movement
     ⓑ reversed film
     ⓒ static electricity
     ⓓ film scratched during processing

119. The artifact exhibited by the radiograph of the *mandibular right premolars* shown below is due to

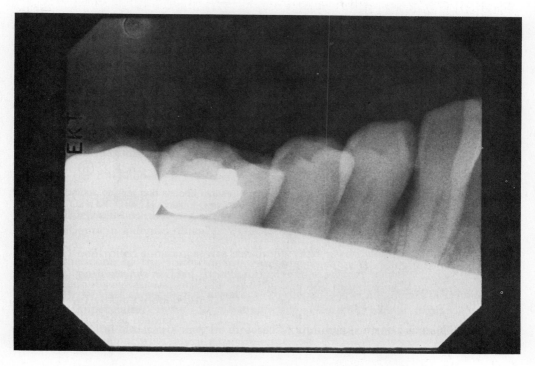

   ⓐ incorrect horizontal angulation

   ⓑ a thyroid shield

   ⓒ level of the developing solution too low

   ⓓ a hemostat

120. One error exhibited by the radiograph of the *maxillary left molars* shown below is

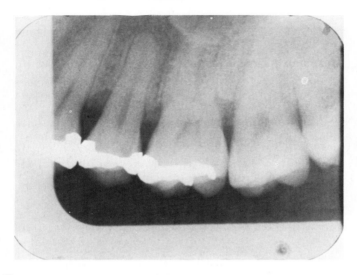

    (a) collimator placed too mesially
    (b) collimator placed too distally
    (c) film placed too high in the palate
    (d) excess vertical angulation

121. The artifacts in the *right molar bitewing* shown below are due to

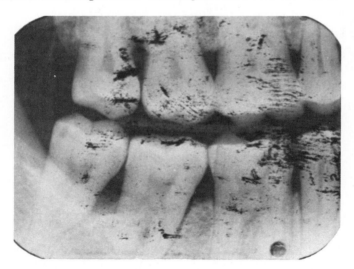

    (1) accidental exposure to light
    (2) dirty processing solutions
    (3) fingerprint
    (4) excessive finger pressure during exposure

(a) 1, 2   (c) 2, 3
(b) 1, 3   (d) 2, 4

122. The error exhibited by the radiograph of the *mandibular right premolars* shown below is due to

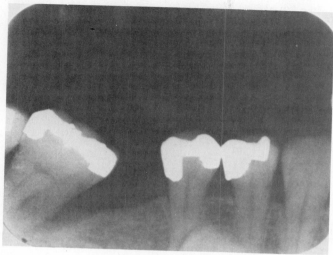

(a) the patient's failure to bite down on the bite block

(b) insufficient vertical angulation

(c) excessive vertical angulation

(d) film placed too far from the alveolus

123. The artifacts shown on the following radiograph of the *mandibular left molars* are due to

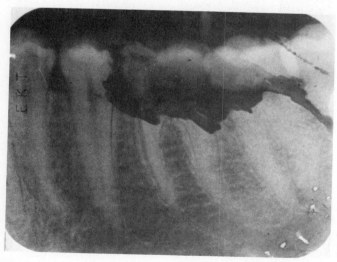

(a) the use of outdated film

(b) developer splash

(c) processing paper stuck to film

(d) dirty developer

124. The artifact exhibited on the following radiograph of the *right premolar* bite-wing is due to

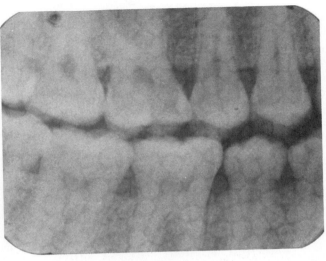

- (a) cold processing solutions
- (b) overwashing
- (c) warm processing solutions
- (d) reverse placement in the mouth

125. The artifact on the *maxillary left molar* radiograph shown below is due to

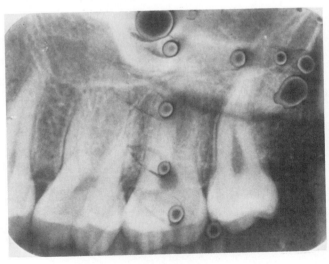

- (a) developer splash
- (b) water splash
- (c) insufficient rinsing
- (d) dirty solutions

Questions 126 through 131 relate to accompanying panoramic radiographs.

126. The error in patient positioning evidenced by the radiograph shown below is

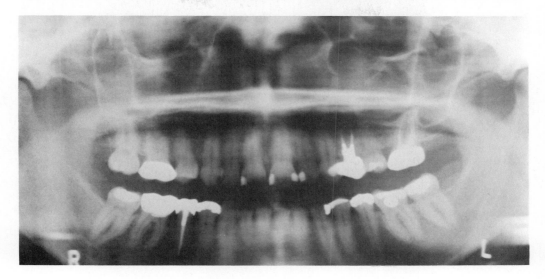

   (a) the occlusal plane is too low
   (b) the occlusal plane is too high
   (c) the head is twisted
   (d) the patient is too far forward

127. The artifact shown on the following radiograph is caused by

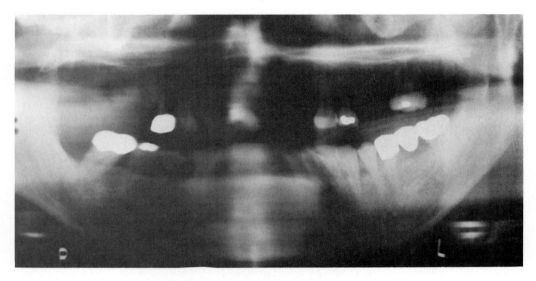

    ⓐ spinal shadow
    ⓑ patient's head twisted
    ⓒ patient sitting too far back
    ⓓ patient's tongue not on the palate

128. The error evidenced on the radiograph shown below is caused by

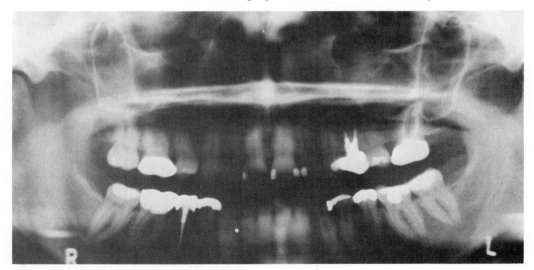

    ⓐ occlusal plane too high
    ⓑ tongue not on the palate
    ⓒ patient movement during exposure
    ⓓ profile index meter improperly set

129. An error evidenced on the following radiograph is caused by

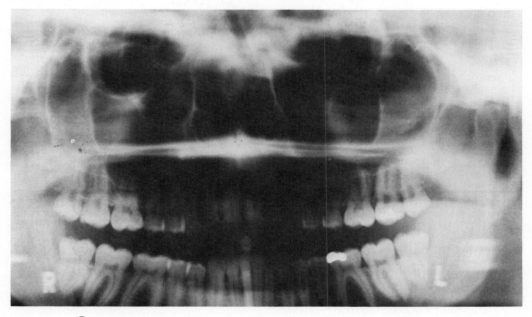

   ⓐ double exposure
   ⓑ occlusal plane too high
   ⓒ patient movement during exposure
   ⓓ patient's tongue not on the palate

130. The error related to film loading evidenced on the following radiograph resulted because the

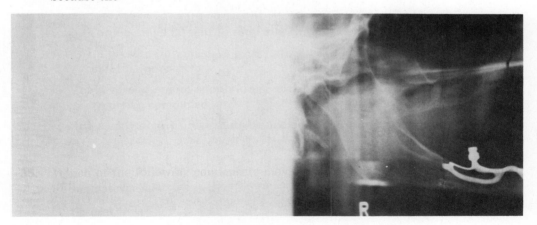

   ⓐ film was light exposed
   ⓑ screens were reversed
   ⓒ cassette arrow was reversed
   ⓓ film end was not at the screen hinge

131. An error evidenced on the radiograph shown below resulted because the

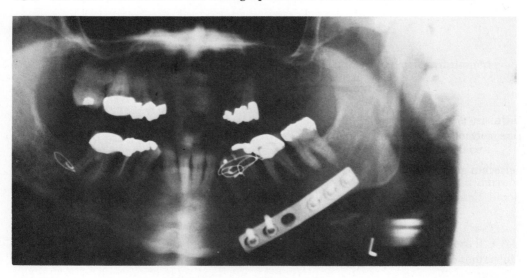

    ⓐ bite guide was not used
    ⓑ chin was not on the chin rest
    ⓒ patient was too far back
    ⓓ patient moved during the exposure

Rationale for Test Questions

TEST III

Rationale for Test Questions
TEST III

ANSWERS AND RATIONALE:

1. (b) X-rays are created when the high-voltage current and free electrons in the tube strike the tungsten target and focal spot. Three conditions must exist for x-rays to be produced: a source of free electrons, high voltage to impart speed to them, and a target that is capable of stopping them.

2. (d) Photons are minute bundles of pure energy that travel at the speed of light.

3. (c) As the free electrons collide with the tungsten target of the anode, the "braking" effect creates x-rays of both short and longer (varying) wavelengths.

4. (c) Another factor in x-ray penetration is wavelength. Extremely dense materials have a high atomic number and thus absorb more x-rays than thin materials with low atomic numbers.

5. (c) Ionization occurs when a change takes place within an atom when electrons are lost or gained and the atom loses its neutrality, becoming either positively or negatively charged.

6. (a) X-ray properties that are useful in dental radiography include high frequency and short wavelength. X-rays have the ability to penetrate matter quickly, thus minimizing radiation exposure to patients.

7. (a) One angstrom unit measures 1/100,000,000 cm. Most wavelengths used in dentistry vary from about 0.1A.0 to a maximum of 1.0A.0.

8. (b) An ion is an electrically charged particle from an atom or a molecule. Atoms that have gained or lost electrons are electrically unstable and are called *ions*.

9. (c) The more dense the anatomic structure, the less dense the image produced (i.e., enamel as opposed to pulpal tissues).

10. (d) According to some scientists, cumulative effects result when exposure is too great and the intervals between exposures are too brief for the body cells to repair themselves.

11. (b) Embryonic and immature cells are more sensitive to ionizing radiation than mature cells of the same tissue. Actively dividing cells are more sensitive than slowly dividing cells.

12. (c) The use of film holders and proper film processing can eliminate retakes and so contribute to radiation hygiene.

13. (a) In dental radiology, the most critical areas in the head and neck are the red bone marrow in the mandible, the lens of the eye, and the thyroid gland. The ALARA principle in x-radiation technique refers to *as low as reasonably achievable*. This principle endorses the use of the lowest possible exposure of the patient (and operator) to x-radiation to produce diagnostically acceptable radiographs.

14. (d) A patient's safety is dependent on the quality of the technique and the use of high-speed film, efficient processing procedures, and equipment of maximum efficiency.

15. (d) Personnel monitoring requires staff members to wear a device that measures the amount of radiation they are receiving. Film badges and ion chambers are accurate and economical and are easily worn in a dental office.

16. (b) Through the years there has been a constant downward revision of the acceptable limits of whole-body radiation exposure, which are about 700 times smaller than in 1902. Occupationally exposed workers now must receive no more than 5 rems per calendar year.

17. (a) The 5-rem yearly limit for radiation workers does not apply to persons younger than 18 years or workers who are pregnant. It is suggested that 0.5 rem be their maximum permissible dose (MPD).

18. (d) Protective barriers of radiation-absorbing materials to enclose the operatory are very important. Lead is a superior material for a radiation barrier.

19. (d) A lead apron and correct technique that minimizes retakes are very important.

20. (d) X-rays are a part of a spectrum of electromagnetic radiation, and their unique properties include the ability to penetrate matter, produce a latent image, produce fluorescence in some materials, and produce ionization of matter.

21. (c) One kilovolt equals 1,000 volts. Dental x-ray machines have fixed electrical output levels measured in kilovolts, which can range from 50 to 100 kV. X-rays produced by higher kilovoltage are more penetrating and have a shorter wavelength. Therefore, varying the kilovoltage of x-rays varies their quality.

22. (c) The quality of radiation produced is related to kilovoltage. The more the kilovoltage is increased, the shorter the wavelength and the higher the energy and penetrating power of the x-ray photons produced.

23. (c) The milliamperage of a dental x-ray machine is a measure of the electrical current that passes through the tungsten filament. The higher the current, the higher the temperature of the filament (cathode) and the greater the number of electrons available for x-ray production.

24. (a) The *ampere* is a unit or quantity of electrical current. A milliampere is 1/1,000 of an ampere (mA). The longer the time of exposure, the greater the number of x-rays produced. It is a general practice to combine milliamperage and exposure into a common factor—milliampere-seconds (mAs). Milliamperage multiplied by exposure time results in milliampere-seconds.

25. (c)

26. (d) A collimator is a lead disk with a small opening that restricts the size of the x-ray beam as it exits the tube head. The restriction of the beam diameter is approximately 2 3/4 inches at the skin surface.

27. (c) The lead collimator controls the size of the x-ray beam at the aperture (opening) as the beam is emitted from the head of the x-ray machine, and it aids in eliminating nonuseful radiation.

28. (b) A position indicator device (PID) may also be lead lined to provide further collimation, and a the 12- to 16-inch PID better reduces exposure to patients than an 8-inch PID because there is less divergence of the beam.

29. (a) The PID directs the useful beam from the aperture in the collimator to the target, the patient's teeth. The PID is either circular or rectangular and has leaded scatter guards built into the plastic or metal extension. A PID with lead linings directs and limits the pattern of radiation.

30. (a) Pointed plastic cones are not recommended as PIDs because the x-rays interact with the plastic and increase the amount of scatter radiation produced.

31. (a) It is preferable for an operator to stand behind a lead barrier, but if one is not available, he or she should stand at least 6 feet away from the patient and in an area that is 90° to 135° to the primary beam. These are areas of minimum scatter radiation.

32. (b) Radiation hygiene protocol indicates the use of lead-lined aprons for the gonadal area and lead-lined cervical collars for the thyroid and parathyroid glands, when they will not interfere with the exposure. The film is stabilized in the holder and *not* held by hand.

33. (d) If no lead barrier is available, an operator should stand at least 6 feet from the patient's head, behind the head of the x-ray machine, and in an area between 90° and 135° to the primary beam.

34. (d) Filters are of absorbing material, usually aluminum, placed in the path of the beam of radiation. Lower-energy x-rays with longer wavelengths are prevented from passing through these filters.

35. (c)

36. (c) Chemicals should be checked daily for quality. A step wedge is a device that when placed over film ("checker films") results in a gradient of gray tones to measure quality control during processing.

37. ⓓ In a darkroom, a dryer equipped with a fan is recommended but not absolutely necessary for manual processing of exposed films.

38. ⓑ Automatic processors can shorten processing time of 50 to 60 minutes to as little as 4 to 5 minutes while producing consistently good end results if the equipment and chemicals are properly maintained. Because total time is reduced, temperatures of the solutions must be increased. Sulfate compounds are also added to the developer to minimize swelling of the emulsion.

39. ⓑ Underexposure of the film can also cause a processed radiograph to be too light.

40. ⓑ Radiographs appearing yellowish or brownish are the result of use of exhausted developer, incomplete fixing, and incomplete and insufficient washing.

41. ⓑ Errors in the darkroom immediately before processing can be attributed to splashing unwrapped exposed film with fixer, water, or developer, causing spots on developed radiographs. The errors may be serious enough to warrant retakes of a radiograph if the spots interfere with radiographic diagnosis.

42. ⓓ The degree of darkness of an x-ray depends on the amount of radiation reaching the film (either the quality or quantity), the patient–film distance and the subject thickness.

43. ⓐ Fogged films usually appear almost uniformly gray, thus reducing the film's contrast. Fog may be caused by improper safelighting in the darkroom, film storage in a warm or hot environment, out-of-date film, and exposure to radiation or light.

44. ⓑ Wet dental film may be read under a white light after being developed for 5 minutes and fixed for 3 minutes. Films should then be placed in the water bath and in this case, fixing should total 10 minutes after viewing.

45. ⓑ The anterior edge of the cylinder should extend slightly beyond the anterior edge of the film. Cone cuts are not always of a semilunar design but may have straight edges if a rectangular collimator (PID) is used.

46. ⓑ It would also be appropriate to include the operator's name on the film mount of a complete radiographic survey.

47. ⓒ If one or more films of a complete dental survey appear clear after processing, chances are that those clear films were never exposed to radiation. As a result, all emulsion came off the base of the film during processing.

48. ⓓ X-ray film is least sensitive to yellow or red light. Extraoral films are more sensitive to some colors than are intraoral films. The distance from the work area to the light must also be considered, as must whether the lighting is direct or indirect.

49. (a) The height and type of the safelight in a darkroom depend on the type of film used. The average height of a safelight is approximately 4 feet minimum distance from the film.

50. (e) Proper exposure, processing, and handling techniques must be used to reduce radiation exposure to patients.

51. (b) The filter and collimator are positioned in the PID attachment to the head of the machine are not part of the x-ray tube.

52. (a) When the tungsten filament of the cathode is heated, many electrons are liberated. These electrons are "boiled off" the cathode and are drawn at high speed toward the target (the anode), where they collide, producing electrons (x-rays).

53. (a) The higher the kilovoltage (a unit of electromotive force that drives the electric current through the circuit), the greater the penetrating power of the x-rays produced (short wavelength).

54. (b) In addition to replenishing the developer, changing the chemicals completely on a regular basis is necessary.

55. (b) A rigid schedule of replenishment is even more critical for automatic processors than for the manual types. Solutions should be changed every 2 to 6 weeks, depending on rate of use and the frequency of replenishment.

56. (d) Contrast may be defined as the difference between the shades of gray.

57. (c) Increasing the milliamperage increases the number or quantity of x-rays. Milliamperage plus exposure time equals milliampere-seconds.

58. (b) X-rays leave the target at the speed of light in all directions. Most are absorbed by the oil in the tube. One percent exit the tube head through the collimated opening and move toward the patient at the speed of light.

59. (b) The main factor in determining film speed is the size of the silver halide crystals in the emulsion—the larger the grains, the faster the film speed.

60. (e) When placing dental film for periapical radiographs, the embossed dot is located above the occlusal and incisal surfaces of the teeth. An exception is the bitewing, for which the embossed dot is directed toward the apices.

61. (a) The vertical angle of the x-ray beam should be perpendicular to the film and to the long axes of the teeth.

62. (c) Horizontal angulation is directed to "open" the contacts of two adjacent teeth in the arch.

63. (c) Exposure time and milliamperage control the number of x-rays only; therefore, most of their impact is on the density of the film image.

64. ⓑ If a film packet is positioned backward in the oral cavity, the film is underexposed because the lead foil situated toward the PID stopped many of the x-rays. Its surface is also the cause of the herringbone effect.

65. ⓑ To eliminate overlapping and to open the contact area, the PID should be directed more distally.

66. ⓑ The beam should pass through the embrasure between the two teeth under examination.

67. ⓓ Minor movement of the tube head is not discernible on a radiograph, but movement of the patient or film results in a blurred image.

68. ⓑ When vertical angulation is too steep, foreshortening results.

69. ⓑ To open the contacts between the first premolar and the cuspid, the horizontal angulation is adjusted slightly distally.

70. ⓒ Using a #2 film, the distal portion of both the maxillary and mandibular second premolar and the molars should be seen on the radiograph.

71. ⓒ Placing the film farther back in the mouth helps to ensure that the film sits in the floor of the mouth and does not extend too far above the incisal edges. Ideally, it should not extend more than 2 mm above the incisal edge.

72. ⓐ The distal oblique angle for exposure of the maxillary third molar area provides a radiograph of the area posterior to the third molar and a view of the second and first molars. Chances are that the second and first molars are overlapped from the distal angulation.

73. ⓑ In the bisecting of the angle technique, the film is placed directly against the teeth to be radiographed, as opposed to the paralleling technique, in which the film is placed away from the long axis of the teeth.

74. ⓒ Occlusal radiographs are frequently used to locate the position of foreign bodies, particularly as they relate to the normal tissues of the mandible or maxilla.

75. ⓒ Either the long or short dimension of the film is placed across the mouth. Any length of PID may be used.

76. ⓓ Films should be fixed for 3 minutes before they are read, and then they should be replaced in the fixer for 7 minutes longer before placing in the final water bath. Slight overdevelopment does not affect film density; however, underdevelopment does. In addition, several other exposure and processing factors can cause films with too light or too dark an image.

77. ⓐ A panographic film is also a choice for an edentulous patient. Because there are no teeth, bitewings are unnecessary, and because the bone is thinner and there are no teeth, the exposure time should be decreased by approximately one-fourth of normal.

78. (b) Maxillary periapical radiographs should show 5 mm (1/2 inch) margin beyond the apices of the teeth. Lack of sufficient area beyond the apical areas of the roots is caused by improper film placement (i.e., film not placed parallel with the long axis to the teeth or deep enough into the palatal area). Also, the film should be placed as far as possible away from the teeth to achieve parallelism with the long axis of the teeth.

79. (c) Kilovoltage controls the penetrating power of the central beam of an x-ray machine.

80. (b) The nonenergized and underdeveloped crystals are removed from the emulsion as the energized crystals of the exposed film are fixed.

81. (c) To ensure proper time and temperature, an accurate means for measuring the temperature of the solutions with a mercury thermometer and an accurate timer are necessary.

82. (c) Keeping a finger between the film and the alveolus when placing a bitewing contributes to proper film placement as well as a patient's comfort because the film does not cut into the alveolus if it is placed away from the teeth.

83. (c) When exposing panoramic film, the patient's head should be tilted downward so that the tragus-ala line is 5° down and forward.

84. (d) Film exposure is not affected by the type of PID used (circular or rectangular shape) on the opening of the collimator or the target film distance. The variables determining film exposure time are density of the bone structure, type of film speed, milliamperage, and kilovoltage.

85. (c) Federal regulation dictates the size of the aperture of the collimator so that the beam size does not exceed 2 3/4 inches (7 cm) at the surface of the patient's skin.

86. (c) A lead-lined PID provides secondary collimation.

87. (b) Film contrast is dependent on three factors: the type of film used, the processing of the exposed film, and the density of the film. A processing time that is too long darkens the radiograph, thus affecting the contrast. Film type applies largely to extraoral x-ray films.

88. (b) Marks on a radiograph also decrease the diagnostic value.

89. (b) The paralleling periapical technique requires some form of film holder to hold the film parallel to and away from the teeth as the central beam of radiation is directed at right angles toward the teeth and the film.

90. (c) In edentulous patients, the parallel technique actually gives the best results if it can be used. The difficulty is stabilizing the film and film holders.

91. (d) For endodontic radiographs to be of diagnostic quality, the tooth must be centered, at least 5 mm of the alveolus must be represented beyond the

apex, and the image must be anatomically correct. A true projection of an endodontically treated canal of a tooth is essential in a radiograph.

92. ⓒ Intensifying screens fluoresce when x-rays strike them, and this light from the screens aids in exposing the x-ray film. The process amplifies the action of the x-rays so that fewer x-rays are needed.

93. ⓑ Dust on an intensifying screen prevents light from reaching the film, resulting in less density on the film

94. ⓑ Intensifying screens should be frequently cleaned using a lint-free cloth and an antistatic compound. The screens and cassettes should be allowed to dry thoroughly before loading them with film.

95. ⓑ Duplicating film becomes lighter with increased exposure to light, and duplication is performed in darkroom under a safelight.

96. ⓒ A patient's consent may be implied or expressed, but expressed consent is recommended.

97. ⓑ The clinician has primary custodial rights to patients' records, but patients have property rights.

98. ⓓ Duplication is performed in the darkroom, where radiographs are placed on the duplicator; duplicating film is placed on top, with the emulsion side toward the radiograph.

99. ◯ **a:** maxillary right molar area; **b:** maxillary right premolar area; **c:** maxillary right cuspid; **d:** maxillary centrals/laterals; **e:** maxillary left cuspid; **f:** maxillary left premolar area; **g:** maxillary left molar area; **h:** right molar bitewing; **i:** right premolar bitewing; **j:** left premolar bitewing; **k:** left molar bitewing; **l:** mandibular right molar area; **m:** mandibular right premolar area; **n:** mandibular right cuspid; **o:** mandibular centrals/laterals; **p:** mandibular left cuspid; **q:** mandibular left premolar area; **r:** mandibular left molar area. As mounted radiographs are held for viewing, the embossed dot is raised from the surface of the radiograph toward the operator; the dot verifies the quadrant and the left or right half of the patient's oral cavity (the operator's right is the patient's left).

100. ⓓ Both the maxillary right first molar and mandibular right first molar are missing. If there is a problem identifying teeth, use the bitewings as well as the periapical films to help in tooth recognition.

101. ⓓ Several occlusal fillings can be seen in this radiographic survey. The maxillary right second molar, the maxillary left first and second molars, and the mandibular right and left second molars all exhibit occlusal fillings.

102. ⓑ Although the right premolar bitewing shows that the contacts between the premolars are open, it is a bit dense for clear visualization, as is the molar bitewing.

103. (b) The mandibular left first molar is missing the mesial portion of the crown. Note the abscesses around both root apices.

104. (b) In this radiograph, it may be seen that all centrals, laterals, and first molars are erupted; however, the cuspids and premolars are not. Maxillary cuspids and premolars erupt between the ages of 10 and 12 years, whereas the same teeth on the mandible erupt between the ages of 9 and 12 years. As can be seen, these have not yet erupted.

105. (b) Although several primary teeth have been filled, the mandibular right first molar also exhibits an occlusal filling. Caries activity can also be noted on the mesial surface of that tooth.

106. (c) As noted before, all permanent centrals, laterals, and first molars have erupted.

107. (b) In the radiograph shown in the question, PID placement is distal and slightly low, as indicated by the cone cut. Film placement is distal, as evidenced by the fact that the entire first premolar and the distal surface of the cuspid are not in view.

108. (d) Errors seen on this radiograph of the mandibular right cuspid include inadequate vertical angulation, as evidenced by the elongated image; too low PID placement, as evidenced by the cone cut; and a processing artifact, which can be seen as a common dark area on the mesial side of the film.

109. (c) Errors exhibited on the radiograph of the maxillary right cuspid include excessive positive vertical angulation, which has caused foreshortening of the teeth, and improperly placing the film too high in the palate, thus not achieving an image of the tooth crowns. Film placement is also too distal, as evidenced by the fact that the cuspid is not centered on the film.

110. (d) The artifact exhibited on the radiograph of the maxillary right cuspid shown in question 109 may be seen as a dark mark on the crown of the second premolar, which was caused by the packet's identification mark.

111. (a) The problems that may be seen on this left molar bitewing are that the horizontal angulation is too distal, with the result that the contact areas are not clearly open and the patient has not made full contact with the bitewing tab.

112. (a) The errors exhibited on the radiograph of the mandibular right premolars can be seen as a light image, which could be caused by insufficient exposure as well as a faulty processing technique and the fact that the mesial of the first premolar and the distal of the cuspid are missing, which is a result of too distal a film placement.

113. (c) The error seen in the right molar bitewing is blurring due to the patient's movement. Because the film is in the patient's mouth, this form of movement is much more obvious than tube head movement.

114. ⓑ The problem noted on the radiograph of the mandibular left molars is due to film overlap during the automatic processing procedure.

115. ⓐ The artifact exhibited on the radiograph of the maxillary left premolars is a cone cut by a rectangular collimator caused by the PID being placed too far mesially.

116. ⓓ The errors exhibited on this radiograph of the mandibular left premolars are that the film is placed too far distally, as may be realized when it is noted that with both molars fully in evidence there is no room for both premolars and the distal of the cuspid. Also, the film is placed too deep in the lingual vault so that the crowns are positioned too occlusally. The black area is due to faulty processing such as film developing.

117. ⓓ The artifacts seen on this radiograph of the maxillary left premolars are due to dirty processing solutions, which cause debris to cling to the film.

118. ⓓ The artifact on this left premolar bitewing is the vertical black line, which is due to pressure on the emulsion. Bending or creasing a film to aid in a patient's comfort causes the same type of mark (usually at the corners). Fingernail pressure also causes a dark line.

119. ⓑ The artifact on this radiograph of the mandibular right premolars is due to a thyroid shield, projected by faulty PID placement.

120. ⓑ One of the errors exhibited on this radiograph of the maxillary left molars is that the cone cuts are due to misplacement of a rectangular PID. It is too high and too distal. The film placement is too far mesially for a molar film, and it should be placed higher in the palate for a clear view of the root apices.

121. ⓒ The artifacts exhibited on this right molar bitewing are due to fingerprints and dirty processing solution.

122. ⓐ The error seen on this radiograph of the mandibular right premolars is due to the fact that the patient did not fully bite down on the bite block. This makes it almost impossible to show the root apices.

123. ⓑ The artifact on this mandibular left molar film is due to developer splash, which results in a dark stain. Fixer dropped on an unprocessed film causes a white mark. Yellow or brown stains on a radiograph are often a sign of improper washing or cleaning of the fixer from the film.

124. ⓒ The artifact on this right premolar bitewing film is called *reticulation* and is due to excessively warm processing solutions.

125. ⓐ This film of the maxillary left molars has been splashed with developing solution. Some water stains are dark but translucent because they just dilute the film emulsion and allow it to run.

126. (a) In the radiograph shown in the question, the occlusal plane is too low, as may be noted by the inward tilting of the condyles. Also, the lower anteriors are foreshortened and appear blurred.

127. (b) The patient's head is twisted, as may be seen by following the inferior border of the mandible from left to right on the radiograph. Teeth on the right side appear wide and have overlapping of the contacts, whereas teeth on the left side appear more narrow. Also, the rami and condyles differ in size. Twisting causes the mandible to fall outside the image layer, with one side in front and the other behind. The problem lies with the alignment of the midsagittal plane.

128. (b) The tongue is not on the palate, and the lips are open, as indicated by the extremely dark areas superimposed on the anterior crowns and the dark shadow in the maxilla below the palate, which obscures the maxillary apices. The patient must place the tongue fully against the roof of the mouth and hold it there during exposure.

129. (c) The patient's movement is evidenced by the part of the image that is blurred and by the film's lack of sharpness.

130. (d) When only a portion of the film is exposed, the cause is usually incorrect positioning of the film cassette carriage of drum in the starting position or not correctly placing the cassette on the drum.

131. (c) The error in the radiograph resulted because the patient was positioned too far back and was also slightly twisted. Anterior teeth of both arches are out of focus and are blurred. Excessive ghosting of the mandible is also seen.

Bibliography

Books

Babbush CA: Dental Implants: Principles and Practices. Philadelphia, WB Saunders, 1991.
Barsh LI: Dental Treatment Planning for the Adult Patient. Philadelphia, WB Saunders, 1981.
Baum L, Phillips RW, Lund MR: Textbook of Operative Dentistry. Philadelphia, WB Saunders, 1985.
Carranza FA: Glickman's Clinical Periodontology, 7th ed. Philadelphia, WB Saunders, 1990.
Carranza FA, Perry DA: Clinical Periodontology for the Dental Hygienist. Philadelphia, WB Saunders, 1986.
Dykema RW, Goodacre CJ, Phillips RW: Johnston's Modern Practice in Fixed Prosthodontics, 4th ed. Philadelphia, WB Saunders, 1986.
Ehrlich A, Torres HO: Essentials in Dental Assisting. Philadelphia, WB Saunders, 1992.
Ibsen OAC, Phelan JA: Oral Pathology for the Dental Hygienist. Philadelphia, WB Saunders, 1992.
Jablonski S: Illustrated Dictionary of Dentistry. Philadelphia, WB Saunders, 1982.
Kasle MJ: An Atlas of Dental Radiographic Anatomy, 3rd ed. Philadelphia, WB Saunders, 1989.
Langland OE, Langlais RP, Morris CR: Principles and Practice of Panoramic Radiology. Philadelphia, WB Saunders, 1982.
Levine N: Current Treatment in Dental Practice. Philadelphia, WB Saunders, 1986.
Miles WA, Van Dis ML, Jensen CA, Ferretti AB: Radiographic Imaging for Dental Auxiliaries, 2nd ed. Philadelphia, WB Saunders, 1993.
Moliari JA: Infection Control in a Changing World. Detroit, Department of Biomedical Sciences, University of Detroit Mercy School of Dentistry, 1991.
Nizel AE, Papas AS: Nutrition in Clinical Dentistry, 3rd ed. Philadelphia, WB Saunders, 1989.
Pinkham JR: Pediatric Dentistry: Infancy Through Adolescence. Philadelphia, WB Saunders, 1988.
Reed GM, Sheppard VF: Basic Structures of the Head and Neck. Philadelphia, WB Saunders, 1976.
Regezi JA, Sciubba J: Oral Pathology: Clinical-Pathologic Correlations, 2nd ed. Philadelphia, WB Saunders, 1993.

Striffler DF, Young WO, Burt BA: Dentistry, Dental Practice and the Community, 3rd ed. Philadelphia, WB Saunders, 1983.
Walton RE, Torabinejad M: Principles and Practice of Endodontics. Philadelphia, WB Saunders, 1989.
Torres HO, Ehrlich A: Modern Dental Assisting, 4th ed. Philadelphia, WB Saunders, 1990

Periodicals

Chee WWL: Considerations for implant overdentures. JADA 20:25–27, 1992.
Christensen: Glass ionomer as a luting material. JADA 120:60–62, 1990.
Clem DS III, Bishop JP: Guided tissue regeneration in periodontal therapy. JADA 19:67–73, 1991.
Clinical Research Associates: Glass Ionomers, Bases and Buildups. Provo, Utah, 1990 (newsletter).
Croll TP: Glass ionomers for infants, children, and adolescents. JADA 120:65–68, 1990.
Donovan TE, Chee WWL: ADA acceptance program for endosseous implants. JADA 20:60–62, 1992.
Kwan JY, Zablotsky MH: Periimplantitis: The ailing implant. JADA 19:51–56, 1991.
Mount GJ: Restorations of eroded areas. JADA 120:31–35, 1990.
Phillips RW: The glass ionomer cement. JADA 120:19, 1990.
Smith DC: Composition and characteristics of glass ionomer cements. JADA 120:20–22, 1990.
Stanley HR: Pulpal responses to ionomer cements: Biological characteristics. JADA 120:25–29, 1990.
Zablotsky MH: The periodontal approaches to implant dentistry. JADA 19:39–43, 1991.